Mental Symptoms in Homoeopathy

Luis Detinis
MD

Translated from *Semiologia Homeopatica* by
J. N. Churchill

BEACONSFIELD PUBLISHERS LTD
Beaconsfield, Bucks, England

© Editorial Albatros S.A.C.I., Buenos Aires, Argentina 1990

This translation © J. N. Churchill 1994

British Library Cataloguing in Publication Data
Detinis, Luis
  Mental Symptoms in Homoeopathy. – (The Beaconsfield
  Homoeopathic Library; Vol. 14)
  I. Title II. Churchill, J. N. III. Series
  615.532

ISBN 0–906584–34–5

Translator's Note: I should like to record my warm thanks to Rosalind Shapiro RSHom and Susana Sutherland RGN, both of whom advised me on the translation of a great many points of detail throughout this book.

J.N.C.

Phototypeset by Gem Graphics, Trenance, Mawgan Porth, Cornwall in 10 on 12 point Times.
Printed in Great Britain at The Alden Press, Oxford.

To my teacher, Tomás Pablo Paschero, with gratitude
To my wife and children, with love
To my friend Hector Vallacco, with appreciation

Contents

Contents

v

Contents

Contents

Contents

Preface

The materia medica constitutes the most precise account of homoeopathic symptoms that we have. Yet the significance of many of these symptoms – the effects of the different remedies on their provers – remains unclear. In what circumstances did they arise, and what were the modalities? Some are left wholly unqualified. Moreover, their pathogenesis in the provers exists in isolation; they have no history.

The clinical materia medicas compiled by the masters of homoeopathy have approached this problem by studying illnesses within the wider context of the case history, based on practical experience. The benefit to our knowledge of the remedies has been enormous.

Nonetheless there remains a pressing need for a greater understanding of the symptoms in the materia medica, and thus of the rubrics that appear in the repertory. It is this need that I address here.

The first half of this book examines the most characteristic mental symptoms in Kent's *Repertory of the Homoeopathic Materia Medica*, 6th Edition. I have chosen to look only at mental symptoms for two reasons: firstly, they occupy the most important place in the hierarchy of symptoms which must be established in constitutional prescribing; and secondly, they are usually harder to understand than general or particular symptoms.

The approach is analytical and interpretative, but in a way which draws heavily on my experience as a practising homoeopath. Practical examples are included under each heading to demonstrate the precise characteristics of the symptoms as they occur in patients. Occasionally problems of meaning arise where Kent uses words in a way which is not immediately clear to the modern reader: 'Malicious', for instance, is taken to mean 'Vengeful'. In such cases I have referred to dictionaries of his time. Each section ends with extracts of materia medica from T. F. Allen's *Encyclopaedia of Pure Materia Medica*, the source material for Kent's work.

The second part of the book consists of six cases taken by way of

1

demonstration at my clinical classes. They are verbatim transcriptions of the initial consultation, and are intended to show how a sound understanding of the mental symptoms in particular can be used effectively in constitutional prescribing.

It is difficult to study symptoms in isolation since they always form part of a whole. In most cases they link up and interrelate harmoniously to present a coherent picture with a complete outline. For example, patients may present associated symptoms such as want of self-confidence, indecision, shyness, and complaints from anticipation; jealousy together with a feeling of being forsaken; affection, compassion and sentimentality, or pride with selfishness and contempt. The case studies illustrate this point.

The book is thus intended to be both a guide to the homoeopath who must translate his patients' words into the terms used in the repertory, and a body of source material from the materia medica which could then form the basis of further research.

Lastly, we should not forget that the most important aspects of homoeopathy are knowing how to question our patients, how to hierarchise the symptoms, and – more important even than finding the simillimum – knowing which changes in the patient indicate that he or she is getting better.

Luis Detinis
Buenos Aires

Introduction

THE IMPORTANCE OF THE MENTAL SYMPTOMS

In the section of the *Repertory* entitled 'Use of the Repertory', Kent makes the following points:

'The mental symptoms must first be worked out by the usual form until the remedies best suited to (the patient's) mental condition are determined . . . When the sum of these has been settled, a group of five or ten remedies, or as many as appear, we are then prepared to compare them and the remedies found related to the remaining symptoms of the case.

'The symptoms that are next most important are those related to the entire man and his entire body, or his blood and fluids; *as sensitive to heat, to cold, to storm, to rest, to night, to day, to time.* They include both symptoms and modalities.

'As many of these as are found, also, in the first group, the mental summary, are to be retained.

'There is no need of writing out the remedies not in the mental group or summary; these symptoms, relating to the whole patient, cannot be omitted with any hope of success.'

Margaret Tyler has pointed out that: 'Kent (following closely as always the teachings of Hahnemann) is very definite about which symptoms are highest in the hierarchy, those symptoms which give the clearest impression of the patient. These are the mental symptoms. If there are clear mental symptoms in the case, then these will be the most important ones. You may find that the patient is insanely jealous or mistrustful, tearful, or indifferent to his loved ones, or reserved, or intolerant of sympathy and consolation.'

And J. H. Allen, in *The Chronic Miasms, Psora and Pseudopsora* says: 'Frequently we hear the remark among physicians, "I have better success, or have greater success, when I base my prescription upon the mental symptoms." . . . Now as the mental, to a great degree, rules over the body, so can we lay great prominence upon a mental miasmatic symptom. This is the reason why Hahnemann gave them such great value, because they were primary or basic, and when a remedy was carefully selected, basing it upon the mental phenomena, the cures were prompt and quite often permanent.'

In paragraph 210 of his *Organon of Medicine**, Hahnemann says: '... Even in so-called physical diseases the emotional and mental state is *always* affected. In all diseases being treated, the psychic condition of the patient should be written down among the totality of the symptoms as one of the most important, if one desires to have a faithful picture of the disease from which to make a successful homoeopathic cure.'

In paragraph 211: 'This is so important that the psychic condition of the patient is often the decisive factor in choosing a homoeopathic remedy, because it is a particularly characteristic symptom.'

And in paragraph 213: 'Therefore one will never cure according to nature – that is, homoeopathically – unless one considers the mental and emotional changes along with the other symptoms in all cases of disease, even acute ones, and unless for treatment one chooses from among the remedies a disease agent that can produce an emotional or mental state *of its own* similar to that of the disease as well as other symptoms similar to those of the disease.'

In his *Lectures on Homoeopathic Materia Medica*, Kent says of Chamomilla: 'It will never cure a sore throat except in these irritable constitutions, such as suffer from pain, such as are easily angered, in a constant fret. The Chamomilla mental state determines when you are to give Chamomilla in sore throat'; and Hahnemann says of Aconite: 'Aconitum Napellus will seldom or *never* cure either quickly or permanently if the disposition is calm and undisturbed.'

Paschero states that 'if the physician understands that the symptom picture can be expressed in its entirety by the mental symptoms, he will be able to extract the most important clinical symptoms of the disease and he will know what is to be cured in each case of disease.'

UNDERSTANDING THE SYMPTOM

Hahnemann warns us of the dangers of speculative deduction, of interpretations that distort the natural image of the illness. In paragraph 144 he states: 'All conjecture, everything merely asserted or entirely

*All quotations are from the 6th Edition, translated by Künzli, Naudé and Pendleton. Los Angeles, J. P. Tarcher, Inc., 1982

fabricated, must be completely excluded from such a materia medica: everything must be the pure language of nature carefully and honestly interrogated.'

The symptoms taken from the materia medica and from the repertory must resemble the patient's own symptoms as closely as possible. They must also agree with the patient's account of his symptoms. The homoeopath can thus be sure that his interpretation of the case will not be a subjective one.

This form of procedure is not always a guarantee that the patient's words are an accurate reflection of what he really feels. He may, for example, describe himself as impulsive, but on being asked to give examples of his impulsiveness, reveal himself to be impetuous instead.

Deduction can be a useful tool in identifying symptoms, but one must take care not to overstep the mark and fall into the error of conjecture. It is often the case that patients cannot assess themselves objectively, and one must be prepared to distrust what they say. Reading between the lines one can often see that the qualities they claim to have are in fact the very ones they lack. (Nevertheless, it would be wrong automatically to assume that a mother is indifferent to her children when she says that she is overprotective of them.) To be sure, psychology does recognise the existence of a mechanism whereby one attitude masks another, and in some cases this may be so. The homoeopath, however, must prove to his own satisfaction that the hidden symptom is actually present in the patient; the psychological insight must be no more than a means to that end.

In a similar manner, and with the same degree of caution, one might choose to see the psychoanalytical mechanism of displacement at work in a patient who claimed to be scared of dogs. The symptom could be ignored if he once had a similar fear of a stern father, and it was otherwise clear that this was the real issue at stake.

The crucial difference between psychoanalysis and homoeopathy is that the former deals in what is latent, and the latter in what is manifest.

MENTAL SYMPTOMS AND NORMAL CHARACTERISTICS

Symptoms are nothing more than the outward expression of the vital force in a perturbed state. They are pathological by definition. The difference between the characteristics of a healthy person and the mental symptoms he shows when sick is one of degree only. Illness augments, diminishes or distorts qualities already present. The character traits of someone in good health – that is to say, who is well-balanced – are scarcely noticeable, whereas in illness some of them become more acute and are plain to see.

The remedy is thus a caricature of the healthy person. The man is not the remedy picture – the man, as Candegabe says, becomes the remedy picture in disease. The symptom is suffered by the patient, or the symptom produces suffering in a patient who is susceptible to it. He is the slave of his symptoms and his behaviour is conditioned by them; he no longer responds normally to his environment. (Note however that the repertory occasionally contains symptoms that are not strictly speaking pathological, such as dancing, an aptitude for mathematics, or precocity.)

Paschero goes on to elaborate this point: 'It would be correct to say that what we call disease is but an intensified response to life – a crisis of adaptation to circumstances – and that there is no difference whatsoever between a spontaneous cure and a pathological one. As we live so we become cured. Every pathological symptom is a normal physiological process taken to its extreme; pain provides us with a warning that we need to give attention to some bodily dysfunction; inflammation and suppuration are the extreme manifestations of normal leucocyte function; oedema is an increased production of intercellular liquid; fever is an exaggerated response of the normal mechanism for temperature regulation; gangrene and decaying tissue, skin eruptions, perspiration, catarrhs and diarrhoeas are all the release of waste products from normal metabolic processes; hypertrophy is the body's response to the over-use of an organ; a tumour is the result of the over-production of cells; mental illness is the workings of the defence mechanism which tries to make sense of the childhood conflict between primitive impulses and repressive education. All these are manifestations of the normal functioning of the organism, disease being a temporary intensification of normal physiological function, an aspect of life rather than some totally disconnected and alien thing.'

THE SYMPTOMS IN THE VARIOUS REPERTORIES

The most reliable repertory is undoubtedly Kent's. It is an 'organic' repertory in which similar symptoms generally appear under the same heading, or else are cross-referenced to one another. Thus, if we turn to

'Arrogance' and 'Pride' in the section dealing with the mind, we are directed to 'Haughty'; likewise, 'Resentment', 'Vindictive' and 'Spiteful' are grouped under 'Malicious'; and 'Ambition, loss of', is to be found under 'Indolence'. The aim of this is to prevent symptoms from being mistaken for one another (and thus from becoming too exclusive), either because the patient has not expressed himself clearly enough, or because the homoeopath has made an incorrect interpretation. The more slender the distinction between different headings, the greater the risk of confusion. Kent warns us to take care in choosing the right headings, and places cross-references in parentheses; for example: 'Impetuous' (see 'Hurry', 'Impatience'). Kent's cross-references have been retained in this book.

Barthel and Klunker's *Synthetic Repertory* is monumental, up-to-date and very useful. Based on Kent's *Repertory of the Homoeopathic Materia Medica*, it also includes information from other sources and headings from other repertories. It has the disadvantage, therefore, that symptoms are sometimes duplicated under different rubrics. For instance, although the symptom 'Idleness' appears in Kent's *Repertory* under 'Indolence', it features as a rubric in its own right in the *Synthetic Repertory*. Kent combines 'Vanity' and 'Haughty', whereas the *Synthetic Repertory* does not.

Kent's main sources for the *Repertory* and the *Lectures on Homoeopathic Materia Medica* were Hahnemann's *Materia Medica Pura*, Hering's *Guiding Symptoms* and Allen's *Encyclopaedia of Pure Materia Medica*.

Note: The number and roman numeral shown in parentheses after a symptom refer to the page and column where that rubric occurs in Kent's *Repertory*, 6th Edition. Wherever the rubric is drawn instead from Barthel and Klunker's *Synthetic Repertory*, Volume 1, this is stated and the corresponding column number of the reference is given.

ABUSIVE (1/II)

One should consider this symptom in conjunction with the heading 'Cursing' (17/I) in order to distinguish between the two. Both concern verbal attacks on people or things. The abusive person uses rude and insulting words in order to offend others, whereas cursing is the vivid expression of a desire that someone should suffer hurt or harm. It also covers the use of expletives as an expression of surprise or annoyance.

In assessing these symptoms, one must bear in mind the patient's education and background.

Materia Medica

BORAX. Violent; he scolds and swears at trifles.

CUBEBA. Impulse to swear at people, to strike them and spit in their face, even to bite them.

DERRIS PINNATA. He is disposed to strike, and inveighs against his dearest friends.

HYDRASTIS. Forgetfulness (while writing); if I want anything and raise my hand to pick it up, or go after it, will forget, for a few seconds, what was wanted, which would make me very angry and feel like damning and cursing everything and anybody who bothered me in the least.

HYDROPHOBINUM. Offended at everything; gives offensive answers. Inclined to use offensive expressions.

HYOSCYAMUS. Insulting, quarrelsome, disputing.

LILIUM TIGRINUM. While attending a lecture, desire to hit the lecturer, and in the evening desirous of swearing and damning things generally, and to think and speak obscene things; disposed to strike and hit persons; as these feelings came, the uterine pains passed away.

LYCOPODIUM. As if out of her mind, she seeks quarrels, makes unfounded reproaches, is exceedingly violent and strikes those whom she thus insults.

MERCURIUS SOLUBILIS. Morose and mistrustful all day; he treated his associates almost insultingly, and looked upon everybody as his worst enemy.

NITRICUM ACIDUM. Attacks of rage and despair, with curses and imprecations. Inclined to be angry and use insulting expressions.

OENANTHE. Excessive excitement; she talked to herself, swore and blasphemed, while at the same time she was seized with convulsive laughter.

OPUNTIA. In the afternoon, fit of petulance, angry at near relatives, swearing mood, not at all pleased, cannot get over the thought of injuries done by friends.

SARRACENIA. Disposition for excesses, to get angry and speak injurious words.

STRAMONIUM. High delirium, furious, unmanageable, talking in an incoherent manner, and inclining to be abusive in her language; she could not be restrained in one position, but was rolling about the veranda as if she was blind.

VERATRUM ALBUM. Cursing and howling all night and complaining of being stupid, with headache and salivation.

AFFECTIONATE (1/II)

This symptom is not present so frequently as patients claim. This is especially true when parents are describing the character of their young child. Often, for instance, it is only the mother who is the object of affection, or else the child is affectionate to both parents but not all the time. If, however, they tell you that he is always pestering them for a kiss or a cuddle – indeed not just them, but other people too – then one can be sure that the symptom applies. Hahnemann's *Materia Medica Pura* has the modalities 'Embraces' (Crocus and Platinum) and 'Kisses everyone' (Senega and Veratrum Album).

If adult patients claim to be affectionate, one should seek confirmation of this in what they say about their relations with members of their family, with friends and acquaintances, and indeed in how they relate to you – do they seem to be affectionate people? This is the best way to understand the symptom.

Materia Medica

AGARICUS. Talking volubly and respectfully, as if to his parents; returning no direct answers when questioned; alternately sings and is vexed, embraces his companions and kisses their hands. He performs all these actions while affected with a general spasm, more like a trembling than a convulsion.

BORAX. Very cheerful, lively, affectionate, with desire and liking for all work, in the forenoon.

COFFEA TOSTA. Love for family.

CROCUS. At times she is very peevish, and morose to others, and the next moment, wishes to embrace.

HURA BRASILIENSIS. The affections are very active (fifteenth day). During and after the fainting spell, disposed to love everybody, especially those about him; he often thinks of death, but does not fear it; he even feels as though he could die without regret.

HYDRASTIS. Affections active.

IGNATIA. Tender mood, with very clear consciousness.

NUX VOMICA. Extremely tender and gentle mood; music affects him to tears.

OXALICUM ACIDUM. Greater love of his children, in one in whom this feeling was always predominant; a decidedly expressed and clearly distinguishable symptom, not traceable to any other cause.

PHOSPHORUS. Tender mood.

STRAMONIUM. They turned natural fools upon it for several days. One would blow up a feather in the air, another would dart straws at it with great fury; another, stark naked, was sitting in a corner, like a monkey, grinning and making mouths at them; a fourth would fondly kiss and paw his companions and sneer in their faces, with a countenance more antic than a Dutch doll. In this frantic condition they were confined, lest in their folly they should destroy themselves. In eleven days they recovered, unconscious of anything which had passed.

VERATRUM ALBUM. She kisses everybody that comes in her way, before the menses.

ANGER, irascibility (2/I)

This is a common symptom. It is one step up from 'Irritability' (57/II), having an additional tinge of violence to it.

The modalities are useful, one interesting one being 'Anger, absent persons, at' (2/I). A Lycopodium woman told me: 'I often find that I don't react when someone whom I'm talking to says something I don't like, but afterwards, when she's gone, I feel furious and even imagine I'm quarreling with her.' Note also the symptoms 'Quarrelsome, disputes with absent persons' (70/II) and 'Irritability, absent persons, with' (58/II).

Materia Medica

AURUM. He becomes angry while thinking of some absent persons.

KALI CYANATUM. At 7 p.m., while walking out of doors, feeling of crossness; carries on a kind of conversation within himself, as if

quarrelling with someone with whom he had previously disagreed; thinks what he will reply in case certain things are said to him. (This state of mind is really painful; there are occasional remissions of it, and there is really no cause for it.)
LYCOPODIUM. He mentally quarrels with absent persons.

Anger, whether suppressed or not, may act as an exciting cause that provokes many different ailments. If it is not suppressed, the symptom is 'Anger, ailments after, vexation, etc.' (2/I). If it is, however, the *Repertory* gives 'Anger, suppressed from' (2/II). Such statements as 'I bottle up my feelings' or 'I can't express my anger' should not in themselves be taken to indicate the presence of suppressed anger if there are no accompanying mental or physical symptoms.

A useful modality in repertorisation is 'Anger, alternating with quick repentance' (2/II), although as it contains only a small number of remedies it is somewhat risky. Sulphur patients often have this symptom.

Lastly, 'Anger, violent' (3/I) covers those people who react explosively, who say they are 'very touchy', 'like a bear with a sore head' or 'on a short fuse'. This symptom is easily confused with 'Impetuous' (54/I).

ANTICIPATION, complaints from (4/I)

This is a very common symptom. Insecure patients with a dread of failure and people who worry about the future have this symptom, as indeed does anyone who suffers either mentally or physically at the thought of some situation in which they will be required to perform or contribute.

Pre-examination nerves would not ordinarily be considered a symptom, unless they were present to such a degree that they were incapacitating, with fears, diarrhoea, palpitations, sleeplessness, stomach cramps and so on.

Sometimes anticipatory ailments vanish as soon as the task or examination begins: the student who was rigid with fear moments earlier calms down and performs well.

People who sit in the waiting room for an hour before their appointment, or who tell you that they always suffer from insomnia before seeing their doctor or lawyer, or before going on a journey, also suffer from anticipation.

Related Symptoms
'Anxiety, anticipating an engagement' (5/II)
'Anxiety, time is set, if a' (8/II)
'Excitement, anticipating events, when' (40/II)
'Fear, church or opera, when ready to go' (43/II)
'Hurry, time, for the appointed, to arrive' (52/I)

Related Symptoms in the Synthetic Repertory
'Anticipation, stage-fright' (column 54)
'Fear, examination, before' (column 498)

ANXIETY, conscience, of (as if guilty of a crime) (6/I)

This is one of the most valuable symptoms in homoeopathy. When the symptom is marked it is generally the highest-ranking symptom in the repertorisation.

The person who feels guilty suffers a terrible kind of pain, for he carries within him both the person who committed the crime and the person who is punished for it. He constantly relives the painful image of himself in the act of sinning or of making that fatal mistake.

The feeling of guilt involves ideas of transgression, of stigma, of sin and error. The patient chastises himself for some minor mistake or for a sin which he did not commit. There may be accompanying feelings of anxiety, worry and distress. It is interesting to note that in many remedies the sense of guilt is linked with an idea of punishment, as though one were doomed to hell or threatened by disgrace.

Guilt may be a central symptom in cases of melancholy. The patient contemplates suicide, which he considers to be both a solution and a price he must pay. Alternatively, the punishment may involve a rejection of happiness and a self-imposed inability to enjoy himself.

It is very difficult to distinguish this symptom from 'Remorse' (71/II). In the latter there is a feeling of grief and regret after committing the misdemeanour. The sense of remorse must of course be out of proportion to the act committed for it to count as a symptom. If in doubt both symptoms should be combined.

Practical Examples
'I always feel guilty of everything, for instance, if my son isn't doing well at school or if my husband has had a bad day at work. I feel guilty for not having been at the hospital when my mother died, despite

the fact that she died suddenly, just when they were thinking of discharging her.'

'I'm very guilt-ridden. My brother died of a heart attack at a time when we weren't on good terms. I don't know why I still feel guilty. I also feel guilty for not having spent more time with my mother when my father died, although I was just a girl then.'

'Whenever I think about my parents I feel guilty. It's as though I want to ask their forgiveness for anything I might have done to displease them. It all began when I was angry with my mother for sending me off to boarding school.'

'I have a strong feeling of guilt. I feel I will be punished and must atone for something, perhaps through the death of my husband or son.'

A mother told me that one morning her 7-year-old son woke up and said, 'I feel terrible because I threw my food away and there are people who are dying of hunger.' She added that her son was always extremely apologetic.

Materia Medica

ALUMINA. Upon seeing blood, or knives, horrible thoughts throng her mind; she feels, for instance, as though she would commit suicide, although she has the greatest aversion to it.

AURUM. He feels uneasy and uncertain and constantly imagines he neglects something, and deserves reproaches in consequence; he appears to carry this uneasiness about him in his mind, and it deprives him of all energy and perseverance.

CHELIDONIUM. Fretful, depressed, anxious, as if he had committed some evil, which gave him no rest. Becomes frightened at the slightest noise, as if he had not a good conscience.

COBALTUM. Condemned, mean feeling, as though guilty of some deed of which others knew; as if he could not look one in the face.

COCCULUS. Anxiety, as if she had committed a great crime. / Great anxiety, as though he had done some evil.

CYCLAMEN. Extreme sadness, as if he had committed some evil, and had not done his duty. Internal grief and anxiety of conscience, as though he had not done his duty, or had committed a crime.

HYOSCYAMUS. He considers himself a criminal.

IGNATIA. Anxiety, as if he had committed some crime.

MERCURIUS SOLUBILIS. Anxiety and apprehension in the blood; did not know what to do; it seemed as though he had committed a crime; without heat, also with a feeling as though he had no control over his senses, all day.

MYRICA. Awoke in a gloomy state of mind, an unusual condition for him; felt very irritable and had a constant desire to find fault; everything went wrong; looked upon this world as a place not fit to live in any longer; considered himself better than the rest, in the morning; felt very low-spirited; condemned himself for various imaginary faults; complete hypochondria, in the afternoon.

NATRUM MURIATICUM. Anxiety, as if she had done something wrong, with heat and night sweat.

NITRICUM ACIDUM. Anxiety, like palpitation, with nausea, without efforts to vomit, as if she had committed a crime, at night in bed; she could not remain in bed.

PULSATILLA. Nightly anxiety on waking, as if he had committed a crime.

RUTA. Very anxious all day, as though he had done something wrong; if anyone just opened the door he feared that someone had come to arrest him.

SARRACENIA. He is afraid, and reproaches himself; thinks he has committed something wrong, or disgraced the family or his absent friends.

SILICEA. Most excessive scruples of conscience about trifles, as though he had done a great wrong.

THUJA. Sudden rising of dark thoughts causing uneasiness, apprehension of misfortune, with fancied scruples of conscience, and with a distinct sensation as if they came from within the abdomen to the heart with sleeplessness and an internal uneasiness, especially of the lower portion of the back, which compelled him to move constantly. / She fancies that she has committed a sin. / Constant anxiety, as if he had committed a great crime, with forgetfulness and general trembling, even to disturbing sleep.

VERATRUM ALBUM. Anxiety as from a bad conscience, as if he had committed a crime.

ZINCUM. Very uneasy mood, as though he had committed a crime.

ANXIETY, future, about (7/I)

It is important to establish the scope of this symptom. Sometimes one's enquiries reveal that the fear is actually more specific, and properly belongs to another rubric, such as for example, 'Fear, want, of' (47/II). If, however, it refers to two or more future-related fears, then the more general heading will apply.

People who are afraid of the future worry about all the different problems that life may have in store for them in terms of health, money, work, study, love and other relationships. They are in other words preoccupied with their fate. Many patients become excessively wary as a result of a fear of the future and take endless precautions to cover themselves against various risks.

The symptom is commonly accompanied by the symptoms 'Confidence, want of self' (13/II) and 'Fear, happen, something will' (45/II).

Related Symptoms
'Absorbed, as to what would become of him' (1/II)
'Grief, future, for the' (51/I)
'Lamenting, future, about' (61/I)
'Weeping, future, about the' (93/II)

Practical Examples
'I take all sorts of precautions because I'm scared of what might happen.'
'I can't live in the present because I worry about the future. I wonder what will happen to me in three years time when I retire, what my financial position will be, whether I'll be in good health.'
(A female doctor): 'I'm very worried about the future, I'm not sure if I'll still have a practice. I fear that I'll get a cyst and will have to have a hysterectomy.'
'I'm very wary, I'm always trying to anticipate the unexpected, to look into the future.'
'The future scares me. Next year I'm going to university and I worry about how I will get on there. I'm not sure if I'll be able to keep up, I don't know if I can cope.'
'I'm scared of the future and of old age. I worry about my financial position and about not being able to manage by myself.'

Materia Medica
ANACARDIUM. Internal anxiety, which did not leave him any peace; he felt solicitous on account of every trifle, as if it would lead to some great trouble; with apprehension of the future. / Anxious apprehension and thoughtfulness, when meditating over his present and future destiny.

ANTIMONIUM CRUDUM. Anxious reflections about himself, his present and future fate, during the day.

ANTIMONIUM TARTARICUM. The whole time an unusual, noticeable (more to others than to herself) wild gaiety, toward evening; this gave place to fretfulness, peevishness and anxious thoughts about the future; she thinks she will remain in her present condition.

ARNICA. Anxiety about the present and the future.

BRYONIA. Anxiety; he is apprehensive of the future.

CALCAREA ACETICA. Sadness, almost to weeping, with solicitous care for the present and future.

CALCAREA CARBONICA. Dread and anxiety of the future, with fear of consumption.

CICUTA VIROSA. He thought of the future with anxiety, and was constantly sad. Excited, with apprehension concerning the future; everything which could befall him seemed to be dangerous.

CYCLAMEN. Profound reflection concerning the present and future, almost to weeping. / He is absorbed in deep thought; he desires to be alone, and thinks especially about his future state.

DIGITALIS. Anxiety, with great dread of the future, worse about 6 p.m., with sadness and weeping, which bring relief.

DROSERA. He is depressed by the persecutions of others on all sides, and also discouraged and solicitous about the future.

HIPPOMANES. Apprehensiveness, anxiety about the future, in the evening.

HURA BRASILIENSIS. Sadness, melancholy; she thinks despondently of the future.

IODUM. Anxiety and prostration; the patients busy themselves for the most part about the future.

KALI BROMATUM. Depression of mind, during which he experienced the most gloomy ideas relative to his present and future condition, if an opinion could be formed from the signs of distress, such as weeping, moaning, and wringing his hands, which he continued to manifest. Two hours after this he fell asleep, and when he awoke eight hours afterwards was perfectly sane.

PHOSPHORICUM ACIDUM. Sad and solicitous concerning the future.

SOLANUM TUBEROSUM. She is much concerned about her future destiny, which she fancies will be wretched.

SULPHUR. The condition seems very distressing, and she is apprehensive of the future.

SUMBUL. Humour depressed, with despair of the future.

ANXIETY, health, about (7/I)

This symptom is instantly recognisable. Some patients try to hide certain ailments from the doctor, for fear that he might send them to have a test which will confirm their deepest fears that they are suffering from an incurable disease. This patient, however, regularly goes to see his doctor and pesters him to listen to his heart or to have another look at a harmless wart, or to have a blood sample taken. His peace of mind at being reassured that he is in perfect health does not, regrettably, last for long. The whole process is repeated with renewed insistence.

Suggestible people and hypochondriacs also fall into this category. A suggestible person is someone who is devastated or disproportionately affected when told that he is looking out of sorts, or who thinks he is suffering from the same illness as someone else, or who reads about an illness and then believes he has those symptoms. The hypochondriac, on the other hand, is characterised by a tendency to exaggerate real or imaginary ailments. He is constantly preoccupied with his health, and always on the lookout for pains and unusual feelings in all parts of his body. Each day he checks his conjunctiva, pulse, face, etc.

Anxiety about health should not be confused with the symptom 'Anxiety, hypochondriacal' (7/I), which, in the original use of the word, means anxiety combined with sadness. Thus, in the index of T. F. Allen's *Encyclopaedia of Pure Materia Medica* (one of the sources for the *Repertory*), the symptom 'Hypochondriacal' is cross-referenced to 'Sadness'. The same is true in Kent's *Repertory* of the rubric 'Hypochondriacal humour' (52/II).

Practical Examples
(A woman said of her 63-year-old mother): 'If she has the slightest pain she worries that she has cancer. She works herself up into a terrible state. Every day she asks me if she looks well.'
(The wife of one patient said): 'He's a hypochondriac, he's got every illness in the book.'
'I'm very suggestible. If I read about an illness then at once I have all the symptoms.'

Materia Medica
BUFO. He is irritable, anxious about his state of health, with great dread of death.

CALADIUM. He is very apprehensive about his health, and apprehensive and anxious about everything.

COCCULUS. Earnest and little concerned as to his own health; he is very anxious about others' sickness.

CUBEBA. Is much disturbed about his health and social position.

NITRICUM ACIDUM. At once she is taken with a peculiar anguish, runs to her physician, but he is not at home, hires a carriage to drive to the house where she expects to find him; during her ride all the anguish is gone; arrived at home she feels as bad as ever, and feels herself thus forced to drive about the whole day, till all the effects of the Nitric Acid have passed off.

PHOSPHORUS. Discouraged about his health.

PULSATILLA. Anxious solicitude about his health.

SEPIA. Sadness about her health.

SULPHUR. During the proving I was much concerned about my state of health, and feared lest I might really get ill.

AUDACITY (9/I); RASHNESS (71/I)

Although audacity and rashness are not synonymous, I suggest they should be combined for the purposes of repertorisation, since the differences are slight and neither symptom has many remedies. They apply to people who would not hesitate to fight someone stronger than themselves, to walk along a high narrow ledge, or indeed to do anything extremely dangerous.

Practical Examples

'Peter used to jump off armchairs even before he could walk. When he was one he pushed over the television set. He isn't scared of anything.'

'He's very bold, he hasn't got the slightest notion of danger, we call him "kamikaze".' (5-year-old boy)

'He is quite reckless in the face of danger, he doesn't know the meaning of fear.' (6-year-old boy)

'He's rash, he doesn't know what danger is, he acts as though he was trying to commit suicide. Once he jumped right into a deep lake, and another time he walked along the edge of a roof that was four metres above the ground.' (8-year-old boy)

AVARICE (9/I); COVETOUS (17/I); MISERLY (66/I)

Avarice is not socially acceptable and patients will rarely admit to being a miser. The homoeopath may be alerted to it by a relative, or it may be apparent if a patient challenges the consultation fees. The miser always complains that they are too high and protests when they increase.

When the miser has to buy something he walks to the shop in order to save the fare. He haggles over the price and is delighted when he manages to get a discount. He never spends money on things that lose their value; clothes, books, or on basic necessities such as heating and light.

He often relies on the generosity of others. Although he could afford to live a life of ease, he never considers himself to be well-off. He is just as interested in saving a few pennies here and there as in making huge fortunes in his business ventures.

His avarice and covetousness are never satisfied. One patient told me: 'I'm wealthy but it doesn't feel like it; I always worry about saving money.'

This symptom is frequently associated with 'Fear, poverty' (46/II).

Related Symptoms in the Synthetic Repertory
'Ambition' (column 24)
'Bargaining' (column 107)
'Greed, cupidity' (column 565)

Materia Medica
PULSATILLA. Envious, avaricious, unsatisfied, greedy, he would gladly have everything to himself.

BUSINESS, averse to (10/I)

Aversion to business, and by extension, aversion to one's work or job is closely linked with 'Indolence' (55/II). The difference is that in this case one is lazy only when one ought to be working.

CAPRICIOUSNESS (10/I); WANTS something, he knows not what (92/I); REFUSES things asked for (71/I)

This is a normal characteristic in infancy. At this age it would count as a symptom only if it appeared frequently and for long spells. It should be seen in the context of the family background; caution is in order when treating children who have been spoiled by their parents.

Two qualities combine in the capricious person: inconstancy (he desires everything, he does not know what he wants, the object of his desires changes rapidly); and obstinacy (his demands are imperative and insistent). The child who has just been bought a new toy has scarcely left the toyshop when he takes a fancy to something else. Deaf to all reason, he cries, screams, stamps his feet and throws himself to the ground in a tantrum. Nothing short of physical force can induce him to calm down.

The symptom is also present in the child who desires unsuitable things. I remember the case of a 6-year-old boy who demanded to be allowed to drive his father's car every time the family went out. He always ended up getting a smack for his pains.

Materia Medica

CAPSICUM. Capricious; at one time constantly laughing, soon again crying.

CHAMOMILLA. Whining restlessness; the child wants this and that, and when it is given he will not have it, or pushes it from him.

IGNATIA. Desires improper things and cries aloud when they are refused. / If she is refused even gently what she wishes, or if one tries to persuade her, even with gentle, kind words, or if others wish something different from what she wishes, then she cries aloud.

IPECACUANHA. His mind is full of wishes and longings, but he does not know for what.

KALI CARBONICUM. He is obstinate and frequently does not know himself what he wants. / Disagreeable mood; she longs for things with impetuosity; is contented with nothing, is beside herself, and gets into a rage if everything does not go according to her wishes, and frequently does not herself know what she really wishes to have.

PHOSPHORUS. Very capricious, sensitive.

PULSATILLA. The child longs now for this, now for that, even with a good humour. / Extremely capricious and peevish at everything, even at himself.

RHEUM. The child impatiently desires many different things and cries. / Moaning, anxiety, ill-humour.

SARRACENIA. Capricious humour, sometimes good-natured, then irritable.

SPIGGURUS. Inconsistent and capricious mood.

CARRIED, desires to be (10/II)

This symptom is of great value in paediatrics. It should be taken in general as a modality of improvement from mental or physical symptoms (worry, crying, pains, etc.)

Young children often like to be carried. The symptom gains value as the child gets older, and to the extent that the desire to be carried is a spontaneous one, rather than one initiated by adults.

It should also be taken into account in acute cases, especially in children who do not usually ask to be carried.

Related Symptoms
'Quiet, carried, only by being' (70/II)
'Restlessness, in children, relieved by being carried about' (73/II)
'Weeping, is quiet only when carried' (93/I)

Materia Medica
CHAMOMILLA. The child can only be quiet when carried on the arm.
IPECACUANHA. Whining mood, must be carried.

CAUTIOUS (10/II)

This symptom is most readily observed in those children who are always excessively careful when playing games. It is hard to convince them that sledging and climbing trees are not dangerous. A mother said of her 6-year-old son, 'He is terrified at the thought of getting hurt. If I tell him to go and play football he says, 'What if someone kicks the ball at me and I get a nosebleed?' When we bought him a bike he asked, 'What if the safety wheels come off and I fall over?'

Another woman said of her 7-year-old girl: 'Lorena is terribly timid and careful. She's afraid of falling over, of hurting herself, even of crossing the street. Her teacher says that on the playground she always sticks close to the walls for fear of getting knocked down by the boys.'

A symptom that is closely related to 'Cautious' is 'Carefulness' (10/I). Although in some cases there may be a complete overlap of the two symptoms (note that in Boenninghausen's *Repertory* the two are combined), one must take care to distinguish between them. Carefulness would usually apply to precision in carrying out an action.

These concepts are illustrated by their antonyms: the opposite of 'Cautious' is the symptom 'Rashness' (71/I) and that of 'Carefulness' is 'Heedless' (51/II).

CENSORIOUS, Critical (10/II); FAULTFINDING (42/I)

The censorious or faultfinding person is systematically critical of other people, and does not pardon even the slightest faults. He loves to identify shortcomings in other people and to let them know of them. There is more than a little aggression in the critic, who never intends to be of help to the person whose faults he reveals. His criticism is destructive, and he is always ready to censure, but never to praise.

Some people speak ill of others behind their backs. They wait till their friends or companions are absent before criticising them. This symptom is particularly prominent in old age. The old age pensioner who is always carping about the ways of the young and their lack of respect, how men's hair is too long and women's skirts too short, is a stock figure. Nothing seems to escape his criticism.

Remarks such as 'I'm very demanding', or 'I'm a perfectionist' may sometimes reveal a censorious spirit.

Practical Examples

'Yes, I am very critical, I can't stand people's faults and I don't suffer fools gladly. When I don't like something I feel as though I have to speak my mind.'

'I have an eye for people's foibles, and I like to criticise them. I cannot tolerate stupidity.'

'I'm very intolerant, I go over everything with a fine-toothed comb, I notice the bad things but not the good things in people and always point them out.'

'I never approve of people, I always look for defects and flaws, however slight. If I don't like the way my staff dress and behave, then you can be sure I'll let them know. At home I criticise my son for his attitude, and if he answers back, like all young people today seem to, then I simply explode.'

'I cast a very critical eye over my family and colleagues. I'm very meddlesome, I always speak my mind about what I think is or isn't proper. I always seem to be looking for faults in other people and this habit does get me into trouble with people.'

Materia Medica

ARSENICUM. He is vexed about every trifle, and constantly talks about other people's faults. Discontented; has no desire for anything. Very fretful and contented with nothing; she finds fault with everything; every conversation, noise, even the light, is disagreeable to her.

CARLSBAD. Very much disposed to take everything in bad part and to be critical.

KALI CYANATUM. For two days, desire to find fault; crossness almost uncontrollable on entering the room; while the cold open air produces good spirits.

MYRICA. Awoke in a gloomy state of mind, an unusual condition for him; felt very irritable, and had a constant desire to find fault; everything went wrong; looked upon this world as a place not fit to live in any longer; considered himself better than the rest, in the morning; felt very low-spirited; condemned himself for various imaginary faults; complete hypochondria, in the afternoon.

RHUS TOXICODENDRON. Disposition to criticise and find fault, from 7 to 9 p.m.

SAPONINUM. Very irritable; nothing goes right; faultfinding, dissatisfied with everything previously done, no matter how well it was done before; find that close application removes this tendency, but when unoccupied I fall back into the same mood.

SEPIA. She finds fault and desires nothing which others want, accompanied by weeping and heat of face. Nothing suits her; she finds fault with everything.

SILICEA. Whimsical and faultfinding.

SULPHUR. Ill-humoured and faultfinding.

TUSSILAGO FRAGRANS. Complaining mood, finding fault with everything, making spiteful remarks, the nature of which he does not himself recognise, and is astonished that others are offended at them; for this reason, when aware of their character, he remains silent for fear of offending his associates.

VERATRUM ALBUM. He seeks out faults in others and contemplates them.

CHAOTIC (10/II)

The chaotic person is completely without a sense of order. Everything is in a muddle. Try as he might, he cannot sort himself out – he doesn't know where anything is, or what he is supposed to be doing. The symptom should not be confused with the lazy attitude of the husband who leaves all his clothes lying around, knowing that his complaisant wife will put them away for him, nor that of the child who lets his mother tidy up his toys.

People may be chaotic at any age, but the symptom is most frequently encountered in children. Untidy boys are typical. Their shirts hang out of their trousers, their shoelaces are undone and their hair is dishevelled. Their handwriting strays off each line, the pages in their exercise books are dog-eared. They are careless, and are always tripping over things (see 'Heedless' (51/II)). Chaotic housewives cannot lay their hands on anything when they need it. They may take just a few minutes to jumble up a room that they have spent hours tidying.

If patients say that however untidy things are, they ultimately still know where everything is, then one can rule out the symptom. Truly chaotic people are more or less completely confused.

'Idleness' (*Synthetic Repertory*, column 597) and 'Dirtiness' (column 400) are frequently associated with this symptom.

Related Symptoms in the Synthetic Repertory
'Orderly' manner, cannot perform anything in (column 792)
'Untidy' (column 1054)

Practical Examples
(A doctor): 'I'm totally chaotic. I can't even analyse my patients' cases systematically. It's the same with everything else.'
'I'm terribly disorganised. A few days ago I lost my purse. I looked everywhere for it – of course I checked my handbag – and finally my husband found it. It was in my handbag after all.'
'My father-in-law calls me 'Little Miss Chaos' because I'm so disorganised. I can't keep anything tidy. I always leave the top off the toothpaste, I leave my comb lying around. When I go shopping there's always something I forget to buy.'
'I'm terribly disorganised – I forget to keep dentist's appointments, to pay bills, I come home late and leave everything in a mess.'
'I can't keep any kind of order. I lose track of time. My clothes are

always in a mess. My pockets are stuffed with bits of paper reminding me to do things. I never use my diary.'

'I'm not very together – always muddled. There are stacks of documents lying around my office – I'm not organised enough to use a filing cabinet.'

CHILDISH behaviour (11/II)

Childish behaviour is a common symptom that may occur at any age, yet it is frequently overlooked. It should be distinguished from infantilism, a hormonal disorder in which physical development is retarded. Childish behaviour may be due to retarded emotional development, or it may simply involve a regression to the characteristics, attitudes, tastes and verbal and imitative expressions of a child. One woman said of her 6-year-old son: 'Lautaro is childish, he scribbles instead of drawing proper pictures, he never gets dressed by himself, he's just a big baby. He cries like a baby and sometimes talks like one.' (Lautaro has a 9-year-old sister.)

The symptom may be found in adults who admit to being 'big kids', who play like, or with, children, and who have similar tastes (children's books and programmes, sweets, etc.) It should be treated with caution in children who suffer regressions (enuresis, infantile speech) before the birth of a sibling.

The symptom also occurs in patients with an emotional immaturity (Pulsatilla, Ignatia): exaggerated fixation on parental images, need for protection, emotional instability, egoism, jealousy, difficulty in resolving problems, etc.

Childish behaviour should not be confused with 'Imbecility' (53/II), or with 'Idiocy' (53/I), which involve mental disability. 'Imbecility' covers a mental age of between three and seven years, and 'Idiocy' one of not more than three years. (Henri Ey)

Materia Medica

ARGENTUM NITRICUM. Imbecile appearance; he looks at people with a foolish expression, even while conversing with them on some serious subject; he behaves shyly and foolishly, and talks in a childish manner.

CARBONEUM SULPHURATUM. Peculiarly idiotic and childish.

CHLORALUM. From having been a woman of strong will and excellent mental power, she became listless and peevish, childish, indeed, in many things, begging for chloral.

CROCUS. Childish foolishness; silly dementia.

CROTALUS CASCAVELLA. She plays with her fingers like a child.

SENEGA. Cheerful, and childishly playful; a slight cause makes him mad and vehement.

CLAIRVOYANCE (11/II)

Clairvoyance should be differentiated from the other symptoms such as 'Presentiments, premonitions, forebodings, etc.' (Boenninghausen's *Characteristics and Repertory*, (213/II)).

Most authorities agree on the existence of this faculty. It involves a knowledge of past, present and future events without the mediation of the senses. The form in which the symptom most frequently appears is that of foreknowledge, usually of traumatic events such as accidents or the death of a member of the family or a friend.

One must suspect the truthfulness of patients who claim to have had such experiences. Very often this is merely an attempt to impress. One should always ask for examples that would confirm the presence of the symptom. Ideally this should be corroborated by a member of the family. People who are really clairvoyant are usually frightened by this faculty.

Two modalities of the symptom are 'Sleep, dreams, clairvoyant' (1237/I) and 'Sleep, dreams, prophetic' (1242/II), which should be combined for the purposes of repertorisation.

Note also the symptom 'Prophesying' (69/II).

Materia Medica

ACONITUM. Lucid (clairvoyant) vision. (Hahnemann's note explains that he was conscious that his beloved, fifty miles away, was singing a certain piece.)

AGARICUS. Extravagantly exalted fancy, ecstasy, prophecies, making verses.

CROTALUS CASCAVELLA. While in a clairvoyant state, he speaks to someone who does not answer.

COMMUNICATIVE (*Synthetic Repertory*, column 144)

Neither this symptom, nor 'Sociability' (*Synthetic Repertory*, column 933), appears in Kent's *Repertory*. They should be added to it. The communicative person feels a pressing need to communicate with others; he is generally talkative and gregarious. This kind of person can hold intimate conversations with complete strangers. The communicative person is frank, expansive and inquisitive. He rapidly adapts to situations and easily strikes up relations with people.

The sociable person has very similar characteristics, and it is for this reason that I would suggest that both symptoms be combined for the purposes of repertorisation.

Practical Examples

'I'm a terrible gossip, I'll talk about anything.'
'I'm very open, I can't keep a secret.'
'I'm a great one for talking, very sociable. I like visiting people and having people round.'
'My husband says that whenever I go to a party or even a funeral, I'm always the last person to leave; that's because I like talking and being with people.'
(A 50-year-old woman): 'I think I'm much more open than younger women. When I'm feeling down I get desperate for company and I often phone someone.'

Materia Medica

LACHESIS. An unusual inclination to be communicative. Great inclination to be communicative, extraordinarily vivid imagination; therewith extremely impatient at tedious and dry things. Lively and communicative, even with a disagreeable feeling of fullness. Social and communicative.

COMPANY, aversion to, dreads being alone, yet (12/I)

An interesting symptom. This type of person wants to be by himself but is reassured by the knowledge that there is someone else in the house with him. (See also 'Fear, alone, of being'.)

COMPLAINING (12/II); GRUMBLING (51/I)

People who complain often do so without good reason, but they always find someone or something to complain about. Indeed, it matters more that they have an audience than a true cause for complaint. There may also be feelings of anger and annoyance.

The classic grumbler is always moaning. If his train is late, he will bore the other people on the platform with his comments: 'It's an insult to their passengers. It's a sign of disrespect. It's the government's fault for not improving the service. I'll get into trouble for arriving late at work . . .' When you first meet him he seems to be a critic, but in fact he just likes to complain. He knows every grumble in the book.

In the child the symptom is generally expressed as annoyance and reluctance at being asked to do something, expressed by much muttering under the breath.

The symptom is also seen, albeit in a different form, in those people who are constantly telling others of their problems, symptoms and every ache and pain. Sometimes it is the patient's family who has to put up with this slow torture, but often it is the doctor who is plagued by an interminable list of symptoms which the patient phones him about every hour of the day and night.

Practical Examples

'At home they call me Moaning Minnie. I complain when my husband doesn't do the housework, when my children are untidy, or when they don't do the dishes. I always complain because it's the only way I can make them pay attention.'

'I know my family gets bored of hearing about my symptoms, but I can't help it.'

'When I was young they used to call me Citizen Smith; I used to protest about everything, always disagree with everything.'

The patient's wife said, 'He wakes up complaining that he is too hot or too cold, if there's something wrong with him he'll keep on about it all day long. He's a real grumbler.'

Materia Medica

CINA. The child is whining and complaining. Moaning and groaning.

CORALLIUM RUBRUM. Very complaining; he dreads and worries about the pains.

CYCLAMEN. More melancholy than ever; she complained of her weeping mood.

DIGITALIS. Much agitated; continually complaining.

IGNATIA. Unreasonable complaining about too much noise.

MERCURIALIS. She complained of despondency and sadness, and wished to weep.

NABALUS. Irritability of temper, complained of in the evenings.

PHOSPHORICUM ACIDUM. He was constantly complaining about his illness.

SPIRANTHES. Excessive complaining, with sobbing. Complaining mood.

SULPHUR. Moaning and complaining, with wringing of the hands day and night, with much thirst and little appetite, though she swallows her food hastily.

TARENTULA. Paroxysm of insanity; she presses her head and pulls her hair; rests about six minutes, and then she begins again, with restlessness, complaining, and threatening; strikes her head with her hands, scratches herself, does not answer when questioned.

THEA. Excessively irritable and weak, complaining chiefly of empty feeling at the epigastrium.

TUSSILAGO FRAGRANS. Complaining mood, finding fault with everything, making spiteful remarks, the nature of which he does not himself recognise, and is astonished that others are offended at them; for this reason, when aware of their character, he remains silent for fear of offending his associates.

CONFIDENCE, want of self (13/II)

Lack of self-confidence or a feeling of insecurity is an extremely common symptom, and has as a result been studied in depth by psychology and the related disciplines. It is natural to the human condition – every human being lacks self-confidence on occasions. The complete absence of this feeling would suggest the presence of the symptom 'Positiveness' (69/II).

The patient who lacks self-confidence compares himself to other people, often to members of his family, and feels inferior to them and the world in general.

One cannot take it to be a symptom unless the patient is permanently afflicted by this feeling, which will then govern everything from his slightest thoughts and actions to his choice of career.

Insecurity expresses itself in many ways: fear of confronting new situations, taking decisions, of coping with the trials and tribulations of daily life, a dread of ridicule and humiliation and of making mistakes. It is ultimately a fear of failure. Patients may additionally refer to a painfully low self-esteem.

The defects responsible for this feeling may be real or imaginary. One must take into account the degree of actual mental or physical debility present in proportion to the strength of the feeling of inferiority. The wider the gap, the greater its value as a homoeopathic symptom.

Practical Examples
'I'm insecure, I feel I'm not as good as other people, I'm always scared I won't succeed.'
'I have a very low opinion of myself, no strength of character, I feel totally useless. I just can't face anything; even going to the bank or the shops is an ordeal.'
'I don't have much self-esteem, I think I'm ugly and hopeless.'
'I feel inferior to other people, I don't think I'm intelligent.'
'I'm insecure by nature, I'm always comparing myself to other people.'
'I'm pretty insecure, scared of making mistakes.'
'I can't be positive about myself, I don't have the will to take decisions, I'm scared of dealing with people and situations. I don't have any self-esteem, I feel inferior to other people. I'm very insecure.'
'I get panic-stricken at the thought of failure, I keep thinking that everything I do will turn out badly. I feel worthless and insignificant.'
'I try as hard as I can to succeed, I go on courses to improve myself, I don't want to lag behind. When I'm at home I have to be the perfect mother. If I watch the television for a while I feel like a fool. I can't stand mediocrity, I get terribly embarrassed if someone thinks I'm talking rubbish. I seem to have a complex about everything, I've got a real inferiority complex, I'm terribly insecure. I try as hard as I can not to let people see how awful I am'.
'I'm insecure, I don't like people to notice me in case I make a bad impression or say something wrong.'

As is the case with other symptoms that are considered to be antisocial, patients will often try to hide feelings of insecurity. They may also develop a psychological mechanism which compensates for their lack of self-confidence by stimulating feelings of aggression, self-importance, pride, contempt and vanity. One must, however, be certain that this compensatory mechanism is at work before extrapolating back to an originating symptom; sometimes patients will point it out themselves.

The exaggeration of what are perceived to be masculine or feminine aspects of the character in men or women – 'machismo' is an example – and the suppression of their opposites, can stem from a feeling of inferiority, a want of self-confidence or even envy. I have frequently observed that Sepia and Lycopodium women do not use their married names in daily life. One woman said, 'I don't use my married name because I don't belong to anybody', and another woman told me, 'I'm just as good as he is, so why should I use his name? Why don't men take their wife's surname?'

Practical Example
'I'm very sharp-tongued, but I think its a defence mechanism, a way of asserting myself over other people, because I think really I'm quite weak. I tend to either undervalue or overestimate myself. I go from one extreme to the other.'

Related Symptoms
'Delusions, fail, everything will' (25/I)
'Delusions, succeed, that he cannot, does everything wrong' (33/I)
'Fear, undertaking anything' (47/II)
'Succeeds, never' (85/I)
'Undertakes nothing, lest he fail' (91/I)

These are really just aspects of 'Confidence, want of self'. The *Synthetic Repertory* has the symptom 'Fear, failure, of' (column 499) which Kent does not have, but all the remedies in this rubric, with the exception of Arnica, also appear under 'Confidence, want of self', in the *Repertory*.

Materia Medica
ANACARDIUM. He is separated from the whole world, and has so little confidence in himself that he despairs of being able to do that which is required of him. The future appears dangerous to him, as if nothing but misfortune and danger were reserved for him, want of confidence in his strength and despondency.

ANGUSTURA. He has not confidence enough in himself to undertake and perform voluntary motions.

AURUM. Despondent and melancholy, he imagines he cannot succeed in anything. He feels discouraged and despondent; he imagines he does everything wrong, and cannot succeed in anything.

31

BRYONIA. Great sense of insecurity, with mental depression, and apprehension for the future.

IGNATIA. Fearfulness, timidity; she has no confidence in herself, gives up everything.

IODUM. Feels unfitted for everything.

LYCOPODIUM. Indecision and loss of confidence. Loss of confidence in his own vigour.

NATRUM CARBONICUM. Anxiety and restlessness; he thought he could do nothing properly. Fretful and peevish; one can do nothing right.

NATRUM SULPHURICUM. Nothing that she undertakes succeeds well, and she does not know why.

NUX VOMICA. She wishes to accomplish much, but thinks it will not succeed.

SANTONINUM. The best marked symptom was a feeling of profound and most unusual depression, accompanied by so much irresolution and want of confidence – in my own powers as to render me quite unfit for work of any kind.

SPONGIA. She is dissatisfied with what she accomplishes; she cannot rightly help herself at work; she does not succeed.

THEA. A most uncomfortable state of nervousness and want of confidence, relieved by beer.

THERIDION. Despair; want of self-confidence; he gives himself up.

Four symptoms are distinct from, but related to, 'Self-confidence, want of'. They are:
'Anticipation, complaints from' (4/I)
'Helplessness, feeling of' (51/II) (see above)
'Irresolution' (57/I)
'Timidity' (88/II)

CONSCIENTIOUS about trifles (16/I); SCRUPULOUS (78/I)

The conscientious person is the self-confessed perfectionist, meticulous in the extreme, a lover of the pristine. He is way beyond the normal considerations of cleanliness, tidiness and order: these qualities are wildly exaggerated in him. This is the baby who cannot bear to have dirty hands, or see a drawer or door stand open, or find a crumb on the floor. The symptom may be observed when children of this kind are at play.

Arsenicum Album cannot bear to see a picture hang crooked on the wall. Not only do they want to put it straight, but it actually hurts them not to be able to do so.

In Sepia women this symptom is often expressed in a mania for cleanliness, which may be present to such a degree that it causes arguments in the family. One such patient told me: 'They say I'm crazy, because when I'm at someone else's house I'll be doing the dishes, washing the napkins and polishing the floor, even if it's late at night.'

'Scrupulous' (78/I) is cross-referenced to 'Conscientious about trifles'. A scrupulous person has a strong sense of responsibility and duty in all that he does.

Materia Medica

HYOSCYAMUS. He reproaches himself, and has conscientious scruples.
IGNATIA. Finely sensitive mood, delicate conscientiousness.
IODUM. Disposition mild, scrupulous, timid, with blunted sensibilities.

CONSOLATION agg. (16/II)

Aggravation from, or rejection of, consolation is a symptom of great value in the search for the correct remedy.

The different ways in which patients say they react to consolation can often point to other symptoms such as 'Pride' (69/II), 'Affectionate' (4/II), 'Pities herself' (69/II), 'Confidence, want of self' (13/II), 'Forsaken feeling' (7/I), 'Love, ailments, from disappointed' (63/II), and so on (see examples below).

One should not take into account a patient's reacting badly to consolation if the person who is trying to console him is the very one who gave offence in the first place.

According to Foubister, rejection of a hug or other sign of affection is equivalent to 'Consolation agg.'

Practical Examples

'I was never treated with affection, maybe that's why I don't like to be consoled.'
'I won't have it. If I'm sad then I cut myself off and try to solve my problems by myself.'
'I don't like it because I can look after myself.'
'I'm very proud, I don't like to inspire pity.'
'I don't let anyone console me. I always wonder whether they feel sorry for me.'

'I don't like sympathy because I feel as though I'm being pitied.'
'I won't let people console me – it's a sign of weakness.'
'I don't like people feeling sorry for me.'
'I don't like consolation – I feel as though I have to manage for myself.'
'Consolation makes you soft.'
'I don't want to inspire pity. I'd rather people were angry with me than that they felt sorry for me.'
'I feel sorry for myself when people pity me.'
'I wouldn't say that I was completely independent, but I rarely get depressed; I don't allow myself to feel sad.'

Related Symptoms
'Anger, consoled, when' (2/II)
'Irritability, consolation agg.' (59/I)
'Weeping, consolation agg.' (93/II)

Materia Medica
NATRUM MURIATICUM. The more he was consoled, the more he was affected.
SULPHUR. During the day, sad, lachrymose; she weeps if one attempts to console her.

Improvement for being consoled, 'Consolation amel.' (16/II), is a symptom that should be treated with caution. Pierre Schmidt maintains that the symptom applies to cases of physical improvement from consolation, as for example in migraine, sciatica or fever. I believe that it may also apply to mental symptoms, provided that the improvement is marked.

If patients tell you that nothing can console them, this may indicate the presence of the symptom 'Forsaken feeling' (49/I). One patient said, 'I cry even more when someone consoles me because it makes me feel wanted.'

CONTEMPTUOUS (16/II)

The contemptuous person not only belittles other people but also feels superior to them. In his scorn there is indifference, rejection and sometimes even loathing. Some people are misanthropists, and their scorn may even extend to animals.

The symptom is most easily recognisable in racists who despise any racial group to whom they feel superior. Another target for their contempt are mentally handicapped people.

The contemptuous person may be detected as easily by his attitude as by his views.

Practical Examples
(A mother said of her 5-year-old child): 'Alexandra has no respect for the weak and elderly and looks down on them.'

(A 46-year-old bachelor): 'My parents were much less intelligent than me. My father was a dolt. I learnt nothing at all from either of them.' And: 'Military service was very trying because I had to put up with the non-commissioned officers who were real oafs; they were much less well-educated than me but they could still order me around.'

(A widow aged thirty-eight): 'I own a patisserie with twenty employees and I have to deal with them. I tell you, they're not very intelligent.' Later she referred to them as 'those bloody morons'.

CONTRADICT, disposition to (16/II)

Patients will rarely admit to this tendency to take the other side to whatever anyone else says or suggests, and the information usually comes from a friend or a member of the family. It occurs in adults of all ages as well as in children. No significance should be attached to the symptom in children aged between two and four, unless it occurs frequently and for prolonged periods. This phase of opposition and contradiction, the age of the big 'NO!', is a natural period of self-assertion.

CONTRADICTION, is intolerant of (16/II); ANGER, contradiction from (2/II)

This type will not brook the slightest opposition when talking or arguing with someone, nor will he tolerate any difficulty or setback that stands between him and the fulfilment of his wishes.

A person who is intolerant of contradiction is generally a 'squabbler' who will cede to no other opinion, no matter whose it is. He is capable of arguing 'till he's blue in the face', of cheerfully contradicting experts on any subject. It is not a good idea to ask about this symptom directly. These patients almost invariably reply: 'If I'm right, then I'll argue my point, but if anyone proves me wrong, then I'll admit it.' Such a response would of course indicate the presence of the symptom.

Materia Medica

AURUM. If left alone, he sits still, taciturn, apparently melancholy, in a corner by himself; but the slightest contradiction excites his wrath, which he first manifests by disputing and talking a good deal, and afterwards by uttering a few detached words.

CALCAREA PHOSPHORICA. Grows violent if his opinion is differed from or contradicted, so that he is vexed not to have been able to control himself.

CARBONEUM SULPHURATUM. He became extremely irritable, violent, and intolerant of contradiction.

FERRUM. Excited by the slightest opposition; everything irritated or depressed her; even her children's caresses increased her bad temper. Was often rude to those about her, because she hated to see or talk to them, and wanted them to leave her in solitude, which alone was pleasing to her.

GRATIOLA. Fretful, irritated by every contradiction, angry outbreaks, misanthropic, with solicitude about his own health.

HELLEBORUS. Extremely inclined to be irritable, the most trifling thing which goes contrary to his wishes excites anger.

HELONIAS. Previous to taking the remedy I never felt better or more cheerful; soon after taking it there was an entire change in the surrounding circumstances; I soon became irritable and dull; could not endure the least contradiction or accept any suggestions in regard to any subject; all conversation was unpleasant, and what I most desired was to be left alone, reserving to myself the privilege of finding fault with everything around me.

HURA BRASILIENSIS. Irritated by the least opposition.

HYOSCYAMUS. The slightest opposition excites him.

IGNATIA. Slight contradiction makes him ill-humoured and angry. Slight blame or contradiction excites him to anger, and this makes him angry with himself.

LYCOPODIUM. She cannot endure the slightest opposition, and is speedily beside herself from peevishness.

NATRUM CARBONICUM. He is angry, and inclined to fight and strike, and cannot tolerate contradiction.

NATRUM MURIATICUM. Easily vexed, petty, he will not bear opposition, for several evenings.

NUX VOMICA. She cannot tolerate the slightest contradiction or the most gentle persuasion to do differently, which makes her beside herself. He weeps if the least thing is done contrary to his wishes.

TARENTULA. Crying and moaning at the least contradiction; consoling words aggravate. Irritable and cross at the least contradiction.

THUJA. The child is excessively obstinate; on the slightest contradiction it throws itself to the ground in rage and loses its breath.

CONTRARY (16/II)

This is contradiction not just in word but also in deed. A mother may complain that in order to get her child to do anything, she has to tell them to do the opposite: 'Don't put your shoes on' – and the child puts his shoes on. 'Don't sit down at table' – the child sits down. The symptom may also be seen in adolescents who go out too lightly dressed on cold days and too warmly dressed on hot days.

Materia Medica

ANANTHERUM. Quarrelsome and contrary humour, but after being angry he often regrets what he has done.

HEPAR SULPHURIS. Contrary mood, he does not wish to see the members of his own family.

NUX VOMICA. Everything miscarries with him.

COWARDICE (17/I)

Cowardice is a feeling of timidity accompanied by indecision and sometimes a desire to run away.

The cowards's motto is: 'Don't get involved'. He does not dare to face up to problems or take any sort of risk. He is convinced that problems are always insoluble and therefore never tackles them. He squanders opportunities and lets life pass him by, because he has no trust in his own abilities or belief in the possibility of his succeeding.

The coward is the person who always avoided getting into fights when he was at school, even with someone weaker than himself. His student days drag on and he sees people younger than himself overtake him, while he always needs 'just one more year' or 'just one more credit'. He is the eternal fiancé for whom marriage involves a whole new world of responsibilities which he doesn't want to confront. He is the tradesman who doesn't take business risks, preferring the security of his small income. He shrinks back when attacked. Fearing a violent rebuff should he say anything, he holds his tongue. He seems peaceable, but really he is concerned only to save his own skin. What he lacks is what the courageous person has to excess (see 'Courageous' (17/I)).

Materia Medica – Cowardice
CAUSTICUM. Loss of courage.
CUPRUM. Fearful; want of courage.
HYDROCYANIC ACID. Loss of courage.
IPECACUANHA. His courage sinks, and he is extremely inclined to be peevish and ill-humoured.
SEPIA. Total loss of courage.
SULPHUR. Sad, without courage.

Materia Medica – Courageous
BOVISTA. Very courageous and vigorous; he would like to fight with everybody.
IGNATIA. Boldness.
NATRUM CARBONICUM. Resolute, persevering, self-possessed, courageous.
OPIUM. Criminals (in India) lose their fear of death and go courageously to their execution. Great strength, courage, contentment with himself. Sensation of courage with activity, as if he could forcibly accomplish whatever was required without dread or fear, with a peculiar sensation of lustiness.

CRUELTY (17/I); HARDHEARTED (51/I)

These are symptoms which in my experience occur almost exclusively in children. They should be compared with the symptom 'Mischievous'. Though the mischievous person may, like the cruel one, delight in someone else's suffering, he is not a sadist and his intention is merely to amuse. The cruel person, on the other hand, causes great harm to animals and human beings without a second thought.

If a patient reports that he enjoys watching, say, torture scenes on television or in films, this alone would indicate the presence of the symptom. In other words, cruelty does not necessarily involve active participation in causing the suffering. The cruel person is invariably merciless and implacable. Certain children are often cruel to animals; in assessing whether the symptom is actually present one must establish the frequency of such acts, and whether there is a real element of pleasure involved.

I knew of a 2-year-old Platinum girl who dismembered two live chicks with a knife, and a 3-year-old boy who would twist and pinch the feet of small babies.

DANCING (17/I)

This activity must fulfill certain conditions before attaining the status of a symptom. A simple inclination and gift for dancing is not enough; the patient must feel it as a need. Many patients report that dancing makes them feel better both mentally and physically. Some people dance alone in their homes every day. If a girl has special dancing lessons, one should enquire whether this was on her own initiative or on her family's. If it was the girl's choice then the symptom naturally has greater importance.

The symptom can occur in psychiatric conditions.

The most useful modality is that which Paschero has added to the repertory: 'Dancing, children, in', which has the remedies Carcinosin, Fluoricum Acidum and Sepia. Parents of children less than one year old tell in amazement how, though their children cannot yet walk, they move in their cradles in time to the rhythm. Although they cannot yet speak, they seem to ask for music to be played.

One even more curious symptom, also cited by Paschero, is 'Foetal movements, music, with' (Carcinosin). I was able to verify this modality in the case of a girl of two-and-a-half years. Her parents said she was very fond of music and dancing and that this had begun before she was even born. Whenever her mother had listened to music while pregnant, she noted strong movements in her womb.

DECEITFUL (17/II); DUPLICITY (39/I)

The deceiver lies in order to get his own way. Patients will not reveal the existence of the symptom of their own accord; they must be found out.

One may lie without necessarily being deceitful, and likewise commit immoral acts without being essentially immoral, but this person does all of these things with a secret, selfish aim. There are many kinds of deceitful people; unfaithful partners, swindlers, crooks and corrupt officials.

Duplicity denotes a certain poverty of spirit. It is a character trait, a mechanism whereby indifference or praise conceal an underlying attitude of criticism. There is a discrepancy between the apparent and the real. This person is not what he seems: he is a pretender.

Related Symptoms

'Slander, disposition to' (81/I). This is a specific and malicious form of attack.

'Untruthful' (91/I)

Materia Medica

CHLORALUM. From having been a cheerful, upright, exceptionally intelligent and strong-willed woman, she had become morose, deceitful, and imbecile-like in intellect, memory and will.

COCA. Mood changeable, mostly very morose, irresolute, false and deceitful characters.

DROSERA. Restless mood and anxiety the whole day; full of distrust, as if he were dealing with none but false men.

DEFIANT (17/II)

This is disobedience taken one stage further. The defiant person is openly rebellious and scorns all authority. Whereas a disobedient person may act passively, this one is provocative. Not content with refusing to obey orders, he rejects them angrily, even on pain of punishment. One patient told me: 'As a girl I was very disobedient. I used to defy my mother and when she smacked me I said it didn't hurt.'

Materia Medica

BUFO. Defiance, duplicity, spitefulness.

DELUSIONS, imaginations, hallucinations, illusions (20/II)

Delusions form a large and important chapter heading among the mental symptoms in the *Repertory*. They often go right to the heart of the remedies. Illusions, fears and dreams are frequently linked. Natrum Muriaticum, for example, thinks he sees burglars, and he also fears burglars and dreams of them.

The following are the most common delusions:

'Delusions, animals, abdomen are in' (21/I). Patients report sensations of some live thing moving around in their abdomen. The symptom 'Abdomen, alive, sensation of something' (541/I) is more general and should be borne in mind during repertorisation.

'Delusions, behind him, someone is' (30/II). This is a very common delusion. Patients often say that they are scared of the dark, and when one asks them why, they sometimes answer, 'Because in the dark I feel as though there's someone behind me.'

'Delusions, faces, sees, on closing eyes' (25/I). If the faces are horrible: 'Delusions, faces, sees hideous' (25/I).

'Delusions, great person, is' (26/II). These patients suffer from delusions of grandeur or megalomania. They claim to be great inventors or fabulously rich, to be friends with famous politicians or movie stars, etc. A Sulphur patient told me, 'I know I'm a very important person. People come to me for advice because I can solve any problem. I excelled in everything I did – I could have been one of the world's greatest guitarists, but I chose not to. When I went into business I was swindled out of a million dollars. I've got a country house with thirty bedrooms. I hold banquets for three hundred people.'

DELUSIONS persecuted, that he is (30/II)

For the purposes of repertorisation this heading should be combined with 'Delusions, pursued, thought he was' (31/I). Both symptoms belong to what psychiatrists call the 'paranoid structure', or in more serious cases, paranoia. The modalities of these symptoms are different in each patient. In some cases the general heading will be used, while in others the modality may be applied when it appears in a definite form.

Paranoid Structure Symptoms
'Anxiety, pursued when walking, as if' (7/II)
'Delusions, arrested, is about to be' (21/I)
'Delusions, criticised, that she is' (23/I)
'Delusions, enemy, everyone is an' (24/II)
'Delusions, injury, is about to receive' (28/I)
'Delusions, insulted, thinks he is' (28/II)
'Delusions, laughed at, imagines she is' (28/II)
'Delusions, murdered, that he would be' (29/II)
'Delusions, superhuman control, under is' (33/I)

Practical Examples
'For some reason I'm terrified of people in authority – government officials, tax inspectors, policemen and soldiers, or anybody in a uniform.'
'My mother sends out deadly rays to kill me; everybody is after me.'

Materia Medica
CROTALUS CASCAVELLA. He fancies he hears some one walking behind him.
STAPHYSAGRIA. When walking rapidly, it seems as though someone were coming behind him, which causes anxiety and fear, and he is constantly obliged to look around.

DESTRUCTIVENESS (36/I)

This curious symptom should be combined with the synonymous 'Break things, desires to' (10/I). It is found in 'hysterical' adults who break things to vent aggressive impulses. The symptom is more common in children, who break or destroy things, even involuntarily. Neither their shoes nor their clothes last long. None of their toys are in one piece – they like to take them to pieces to see how they work, or to 'mend' them irreparably.

DICTATORIAL (36/I); DOGMATIC (37/I); DOMINEERING (37/I)

The dictatorial, bossy and domineering type of person is well known to everybody. The symptom may appear at a very early age. It is present in the baby who insistently demands attention, and in the child who is excessively independent, who gives orders and imposes his will on those around him. The aim of the dictatorial person is to hold sway over others. Everyone must be at his service and at his disposal.

One may contrast this symptom with the quality of leadership, which is quite normal; some individuals have a natural authority. While the leader puts himself at the service of others or of a cause, the dictator puts the cause or the other people at his own service. Anyone who shows leadership qualities and ability is expelled from the group, because the dictator fears that one day he may himself be ousted.

When applying this symptom to patients who are always trying to have their way, or who demand attention, or want other people to do things for them, one must take care to establish that their behaviour is not due to selfishness or laziness. For example, one Sulphur patient said, 'I enjoy giving orders because I'm lazy and I like other people to do things for me.' Here the symptom is clearly 'Laziness', not 'Dictatorial'.

A Lycopodium patient hid feelings of inferiority behind a dictatorial demeanour. He told me, 'I'm strict because to be weak is a sign of inferiority.'

Kent places 'Dogmatic' (37/I) under the rubric 'Dictatorial', no doubt because this symptom frequently occurs in strong and dominant personalities. The dogmatic person has characteristics that are shared by the symptoms 'Fanaticism' (41/II) and 'Positiveness' (69/II). He upholds extreme points of view and is devoted to utopian ideas. His doctrine admits of no errors, and he attempts to impose it blindly, although its principles may be dubious and even incoherent.

Materia Medica

ARNICA. Sullen insolence and imperiousness.

LYCOPODIUM. Delirious, raging, envious, reproachful, presumptuous, and imperious.

DIRTINESS (*Synthetic Repertory*, column 400)

This symptom does not appear in Kent's *Repertory*.

The dirty person is indifferent and sometimes actually averse to cleanliness. Such children can only be induced to have a bath or brush their teeth by brute force. Some women report that they have the greatest trouble in making their husbands put on a clean shirt.

One can identify this symptom when examining the patient: the navel and the fingernails are dirty, there is body odour, the shirt cuffs are grubby and the shoes unpolished.

Children with this symptom simply cannot stay clean. They roll on the floor, they get dirty when eating. Some are so filthy that they eat their own mucus, or food that is unhygienic (Kent).

The symptom 'Skin Filthy' (1325/I) is of great value. Some babies have visible 'collars of dirt' around their necks, or dirt between the fingers and toes, despite taking frequent baths. They seem to have a magnetic attraction for dirt.

DISOBEDIENCE (37/I)

This is most often found in rebellious children and adolescents, in revolt against authority. They disregard orders and rules.

A mother said of her 5-year-old daughter: 'The best word to describe Laura is 'disobedient', she hasn't got any respect. She won't take no for an answer. She doesn't obey the school rules, she won't listen to the teacher and she does as she pleases.'

The opposite symptom to 'Disobedience' is 'Mildness' 65/II).

Materia Medica
CHINA. Want of docility. Disobedience.
LYCOPODIUM. The child becomes disobedient, though not ill-humoured.
VIOLA TRICOLOR. Disobedience.

DWELLS on past disagreeable occurrences (39/I)

People with this symptom are constantly reliving incidents from the past, predominantly sad ones. They experience accompanying feelings of grief, resentment, guilt, injustice, etc.

The patient dwells on some ancient offence. He turns it over in his mind, his memory keeps it alive, stays faithful to it. In patients with a masochistic character the symptom may be a means of chastising themselves. Kent's *Lectures on the Homoeopathic Materia Medica* shows that this is typical of Natrum Muriaticum: 'Unpleasant occurrences are recalled that she may grieve over them.' One patient told me, 'I dwell on the past and torture myself by thinking about all the bad things I have done.'

Materia Medica

BENZOICUM ACIDUM. The mind is inclined to dwell upon unpleasant things. If he saw anyone who was deformed it made him shudder.

HEPAR SULPHURIS. She remembers everything that has been unpleasant during her life.

LYCOPODIUM. She is overpowered by many unpleasant recollections, about which she becomes vexed; even at night on waking.

MENYANTHES. Despondent mood; his thoughts incline to dwell upon past, sad, disagreeable subjects.

NATRUM MURIATICUM. If she only thinks of a want long since past, tears come into her eyes. / He seemed to seek for past unpleasant occurrences, in order to think them over making himself morbid. / Full of grief; he tormented himself; he seemed to prefer disagreeable thoughts, which prostrated him very much.

SEPIA. The recollection of past unpleasant circumstances puts him in an extreme ill-humour.

SULPHUR. Vexatious and morbid ideas of the past arise from the most indifferent thoughts, and from every occurrence in life, which continue to be united with new vexations so that she cannot free herself from them, together with a courageous mood which is ready for great resolution.

EGOTISM (39/I)

Patients do not easily admit to being egotists. It is as though they were not aware of the symptom. Egotism (and by extension, also self-centredness or self-adoration) is usually mentioned by other people or can be deduced directly.

The egotist does nothing but talk of himself all the time. Every time he opens his mouth he uses the word 'I'. He is obsessed with his body; one may justifiably suspect that the symptom is present whenever a patient appears excessively concerned with himself, describing his symptoms in minute detail and fussing about his health (not to be confused with 'Anxiety, health, about' (7/I)).

A minor fall from a horse, or a small spot that has appeared on his leg, becomes a major issue. He never mentions his family, not even during a casual conversation. His wife may be in hospital, or his son may just have passed an important examination, but he will continue to talk only of himself. He is the sole source of his satisfactions and preoccupations. No one else counts.

Among the characteristics that are always present to a greater or lesser degree in this symptom are vanity, contempt, egotism and coquetry. It is frequently associated with 'Contemptuous' (16/I) and 'Pride' (69/II).

Boredom ENNUI (39/II)

Ennui or boredom is a symptom that occurs in people of all ages, though predominantly in children.

Nothing attracts the attention or arouses the enthusiasm of the person suffering from ennui. He clamours for something to do, something in which to invest his energy, but nothing seems to him to be really worthwhile. His world is a gloomy one in which all tasks are humdrum and all people mediocre. He is never in the right place or in the right company.

Though he does not know how to fill his time, he is acutely aware of its passing, and this is a source of torment for him. The repetitiveness of experience dulls his appetite and exhausts him. Everything seems old and worn. He is paralysed by a feeling of disgust and premature failure. His ennui is a prison cell from which he cannot escape. Life, according to him, is monotonous and featureless. He accepts it only reluctantly.

He differs from the indolent person in that his boredom is a cause of suffering to him. The indolent person merely shrugs his shoulders. Nor is he like the indifferent person who is simply not interested in doing anything. He has the desire to act but does not know how to.

In actual fact, the bored person is not attracted by the world because he no longer looks at it; for him, everything was better in the past. He cannot appreciate what he has today because it is not as good as what he had yesterday. Weighing up his life, he wonders whether it is worth living. But he does not surrender to melancholy or indolence. In a certain sense he is a rebel, demanding and hopeful, although he may also seem querulous and embittered. Ultimately he has simply lost the habit of being cheerful.

The symptom does not refer to people whom others find boring.

Practical Examples

'I'm constantly fed up and bored, I don't want to talk to anyone.'

'Nothing interests me, everything I used to enjoy now bores me.'

(A mother said of her 6-year-old girl): 'All she says is, "What can I do, I'm bored".'

'I'm always bored, I don't know what to do, how to fill my time.'

'I have a great sense of tedium, I feel like a machine. Nothing ever changes, I go to work, take the kids to school, play golf on Sundays. Everything I do bores me – I have no enthusiasm for anything.'

Materia Medica

ALUMINA. Intolerable ennui; an hour seems to him half a day.

CURARE. Constant ennui.

HURA BRASILIENSIS. In general she is careless of the future; ennui and weeping; thinks about death without fearing it.

KALI BICHROMICUM. Discouragement amounting to ennui.

KALI IODATUM. Ennui, lachrymose mood, sad expression.

LACHESIS. Ennui with trembling.

LYCOPODIUM. Ennui.

MAGNESIA MURIATICA. Anxious and apprehensive, with ennui, towards evening.

MANCINELLA. He is bored by everything.

NATRUM CARBONICUM. Ennui; he is absorbed in himself, and does not even know how he is, in the morning.

NUX VOMICA. Ennui; the time seems intolerably long, during the first hours.

PETROLEUM. No desire to work; no pleasure in objects of which he was usually fond, hence intolerable ennui.

SPIRANTHES. Indolence and ennui.

TARENTULA. Ennui, alternating with mirth. / Ennui, crossness, easily made angry, contrary to his habit and disposition.

ZINCUM. Apprehension and ennui; she seeks society.

ENVY (39/II)

Envy is a distressing and rather complex symptom. It combines burning desire for the thing that cannot be had with regret and a feeling of ill-will, or even hatred, for the person who has it. The coveted thing may be a material object or an abstract quality such as talent, power, honour, knowledge, glory, fortune, youth, nobility, or social standing, and so on.

The envious person is constantly comparing himself with others, and this leads him to compete whenever possible with the person he envies. He will buy a car that is larger than his neighbour's, or will have more expensive redecorations done to his house in order to go one better. Even if he did have more than his rival he would still find something to envy in him.

While this is a common kind of feeling, it is difficult to detect during the consultation, unless the homoeopath is particularly observant and asks some searching questions, or else reads between the lines of what the patient says. The patient himself may not even be aware that he is envious.

One of my patients, a bank manager, married with two children, told me: 'It's not that I'm jealous of my son. He's a doctor – a professional – and I'm not . . .' As he did not elaborate, I pressed him to tell me what his feelings were about the fact that his son was a professional. He replied: 'It's not envy, no . . . I just feel proud of him.'

Later, talking of his job, he said: 'No one is as good as I am, or knows as much as I do at the bank. I'm a real professional, I exercise my authority and demand that my staff give of their very best.' It was clear from these words that he did indeed envy his son, despite his protestations to the contrary. He compensated for the frustrated desire to be like his son by making himself a 'professional' at the bank.

Envy should not be confused with emulation, which does not involve feelings of ill-will or hatred. In this case, comparison and competition are not accompanied by painful feelings of inadequacy. There is instead a desire to imitate with a view to improving oneself.

Materia Medica

CURARE. Melancholy egotistical, envious, intractable disposition.

LILIUM TIGRINUM. Symptoms came down on her like a sudden cloud, when she was feeling quite well (thirty-sixth day); she lost vigour and snap, and could sit down and cry, or be impatient with herself and tear about, but feels hurried; could walk or run aimlessly for an indefinite time; with all this depression comes a desire for fine things of all kinds; she is dissatisfied with what she has and is envious of others.

LYCOPODIUM. Delirious, raging, envious, reproachful, presumptuous and imperious.

PULSATILLA. Envious, avaricious, unsatisfied, greedy, he would gladly have everything to himself.

SARRACENIA. Invidious, distrustful, and suspicious character.

FANATICISM (41/II)

'Fanaticism' may be seen in men and women of all ages, but most often in the young. These people may belong to any political party or religious group; hence the importance of finding out about the interests and persuasions of one's patients.

The fanatic may be readily identified by his attitude and behaviour. Within a group he will be passionately enthusiastic in support of an idea. The greater the validity of an objection, the more aggressive and dogged will be his defence of them. He would rather die than admit that he might be wrong and his adversary right. This may lead him to compound his problems to an absurd degree, rather than to try to solve them.

His blindness and lack of flexibility prevent him from clarifying his own thoughts or from exchanging ideas. He shuts himself off from all other points of view.

Fanaticism in children may be recognised by a manic or extreme attachment to something. A mother said of her 6-year-old son: 'He gets crazy about certain things. At one time he used to play with his go-kart all day, now he's dropped everything for football. You can see him on the street kicking his ball around, even kicking stones.'

Religious fanaticism comes under the heading of 'Religious affections' (71/II). One female patient (Sulphur) told me: 'I'm very religious, and feel deeply for Jesus Christ. I think about his teachings all the time – my whole life revolves around religion.'

Materia Medica

THUJA. Weak-minded, with pious fanaticism, dread of work, incessant restlessness, sleeplessness, constipation and suppression of the menses, gradually decreased fourteen days after taking the remedy, and within nine months became permanently and radically cured.

FEAR (42/I)

The *Repertory* contains a large variety of fears, and all are of great value in the search for the simillimum. These are the most common:

FEAR, accidents, of (43/I)

This symptom should not be confused with 'Fear, happen, something will' (45/II). It should be ruled out if the patient or a close friend or relative has suffered a serious accident.

FEAR, alone, of being (43/I)

This is easy enough to understand. If the fear of being alone arises from the fact that in these circumstances the patient is scared of burglars, then its significance diminishes or it may be rejected altogether. (See also 'Company, aversion to, dreads being alone, yet'.)

FEAR, animals, of (43/I)

Most often found in women and children. Applicable when the fear is of all kinds of animals. If the animals concerned are dogs or cats then one should refer to the appropriate heading; 'Fear, dogs, of' (44/II) and 'Fear, cats, of' (*Synthetic Repertory*, column 483). Silica (Paschero) should be added to the latter rubric.

One should rule out a fear of dogs that originated in a traumatic real-life incident, in which the patient was attacked or bitten by a dog. The symptom is of real value only when the patient realises that it is absurd and without any logical basis. For instance, he might be scared of a harmless puppy, or invariably cross the street in order to avoid passing a dog on the pavement.

FEAR, crowd, in a (43/II)

This is the fear felt at football stadiums, cinemas, theatres, demonstrations and other crowded places. It must be differentiated from 'Fear, people, of' (46/II), a symptom in which the number of people present is irrelevant and which usually has to do with feelings of persecution. One patient said, 'People frighten me because they can react very aggressively – they can attack you for no reason at all.'

FEAR, dark (43/II)

Fear of the dark is usual between the ages of two and five. If it is to have any value as a symptom in young children it must therefore be markedly present over a long period of time. One should not take into account fear of the dark in an unknown place, or fear of entering an unlit house. The symptom can also be ignored in children whose parents have accustomed them to sleep with a small light on in their room, or with a chink of light showing through the door. If adult patients cannot go to sleep in a totally dark room then it is definitely present.

The symptom may also be rejected if it transpires that the fear is actually one of ghosts, or if there is a feeling that someone is standing behind one – symptoms that occur in some patients when they are in the dark.

FEAR, death, of (44/I)

This is a natural human fear which only becomes a symptom when it is so strong as to disrupt the normal life of the patient. The fear may be of death in the immediate or distant future. One must enquire as to the cause of the symptom: for example, it would have to be discarded in the case of a jealous patient who admitted that he could not bear the thought of his wife remarrying should he himself die.

FEAR, destination, of being unable to reach his (44/I)

The 'destination' is meant in a literal rather than a metaphorical sense. The cause of this symptom is physical weariness.

Materia Medica
LYCOPODIUM. Weariness and exhaustion while walking so that he feared that he would be unable to reach his destination, at 5 p.m.

FEAR, disease, of impending (44/II)

This rubric refers to any kind of illness that is not imminent. Fear of illness is in many cases associated with fear of death. Patients' replies, on being asked why they are afraid of illness, often throw invaluable light on their characters. One said, 'I'm scared of falling ill because illnesses are disabling and that makes me feel inferior to other people. I always give the impression that I'm well.'

A fear of dogs may conceal a fear of being infected with rabies. Fear of contagious diseases features in the *Synthetic Repertory*: 'Fear, disease, contagious, epidemic diseases, of' (column 494). In Kent's *Repertory* it appears as 'Fear, infection, of' (45/II). Both headings should be combined for the purposes of repertorisation. A patient who worked in a hospital said, 'I worry terribly about catching something. My fear of patients with contagious diseases makes it very hard to do my job properly. I may have to leave.'

Fear of infection can also be expressed as a fear of catching tetanus, epidemic diseases, or contaminating oneself by physical contact with everyday objects (a fear which leads the patient to wash his hands frequently in order to avoid contamination). One patient told me, 'I never touch the handrail in the bus. I'm terrified if someone sneezes or coughs in front of me. I don't go to the bathroom anywhere except at home.'

FEAR, evil, of (44/II)

Two very closely related symptoms are 'Fear, happen, something will' (45/II) and 'Fear, misfortune, of' (46/I). A close analysis of these three symptoms and of the paragraphs in which they are described in Allen's *Encyclopaedia of Pure Materia Medica* suggests that on the whole they all have the same meaning, though it is expressed in different ways by the provers.

Thus, 'Fear, evil, of' almost always appears to mean a fear that some harm may occur. The symptom 'Fear, happen, something will', is again, more specifically, a fear that something bad will happen. I therefore consider that for the purposes of repertorisation, 'Fear, evil of' should be combined with 'Fear, happen, something will' when one is dealing with a patient who has the latter symptom.

The symptom 'Fear, misfortune of' applies when the patient expresses it literally and spontaneously, but one must bear in mind its close relationship with the other two symptoms. In most cases the patient who says he fears something bad is going to happen will, when asked to be more specific, mention a misfortune or accident of some kind.

One woman told me, 'When my husband or one of the children is late coming home I inevitably think that something awful has happened to them. When my daughter had a fever I thought she was going to die, and the same thing happened when my sister had hepatitis.'

Materia Medica – Fear, evil, of

ALUMINA. She is constantly possessed by bad thoughts, which oblige her to weep; at the same time she feels apprehensive and uneasy, as if something evil were to happen to her; everything that she only looks at, fills her with sadness.

ARNICA. Apprehension of future evils.

CALCAREA ACETICA. Anxious disposition, as though something evil were impending or to be dreaded in the future, with constant inclination to work.

CALCAREA CARBONICA. Fearful and restless, as if something evil would happen.

CALCAREA SULPHURICA. Excessive, bitter melancholy, with distressing apprehensions of evil to loved ones.

CASTOREUM. Very melancholy and depressed, as if something evil would befall her, in the afternoon.

CAUSTICUM. Anxious apprehension lest something evil should happen, with urging to stool.

CHININUM SULPHURICUM. The day being clear and windy, and a holiday to many, few people being on the street produced a sort of street-quietness; felt a gloom come over me, as if some evil were impending; relieved by a specific trust in the Almighty; this from 3 to 4.15 p.m. Recurrence of feeling of impending evil, in the afternoon. / Great anxiety, amounting to an apprehension, as if some evil would happen.

CINA. Great anxiety and apprehension, while walking in the open air, as if something evil had happened to him.

CLEMATIS. Anxious uneasiness, as though some evil would befall him.

FERRUM. Anxiety, as if something evil had happened to her. Anxiety at night, as if some evil had happened to her; she could not sleep; tossed about in bed.

KALI IODATUM. Very apprehensive and lachrymose, as if some evil were impending, in the evening, lasting two hours.

LACHESIS. So great appehensiveness while riding in the open air that it seemed to him some great evil was impending, like an evil foreboding; it tormented him for more than an hour.

MENYANTHES. Apprehensive sensation about the heart, as of impending evil, and as if he had to endure some hardship.

Materia Medica – Fear, happen, something will

CAUSTICUM. Great apprehension whenever. anything happens; despondent, depressed, most excessive exhaustion and prostration. Anxious uneasy mood, as if something unpleasant impended; this unfits him for every work.

ELAPS. Fearfulness, dread of being alone, as though something would happen, or as though a rowdy would break in.

FLUORICUM ACIDUM. During the tottering sensation he has a decided though not anxious expectation, as if something awful was to happen there, but he feels no anxiety. / Sensation as if dangers did menace him, but without being afraid; particularly during the pressure in the occiput, during the staggering, the pain in the bladder, etc.

HYDROPHOBINUM. Feeling as if I had heard, or was about to hear something bad; morose and crabbed feelings until 4 p.m. / Mind much depressed; felt as if something disagreeable was about to happen. / Feeling as if something annoying was about to happen; goes off when thinking of it. / He cannot prevent ideas of something awful about to happen, or as if he would do something awful. / An indescribable idea, which I could not shake off, of something dreadful about to happen to me; all day feeling as if some great misfortune were about to occur.

KALMIA. A feeling of anxiety; feel as though something dreadful was going to happen to me.

MOSCHUS. Anxiety, as if something were about to happen.

STRYCHNINUM. A fear of something about to occur.

Materia Medica – Fear, misfortune, of

ANACARDIUM. Illusions of the fancy; he imagines he hears his name called by the voice of his far-distant mother and sister, accompanied by an apprehension of misfortune and anxiety.

ASTERIAS RUBENS. Feeling of excessive anguish from noon till 3 p.m., it seems as if some misfortune was impending, as if he was going to hear bad news, he then feels as if he should give way to tears (sixth day). / Depression, feeling of weariness; it seems as if some misfortune was about to happen to him, and that, should it actually come upon him, he would weep, rather than brace himself to meet it, or become angry.

CALCAREA CARBONICA. Frightened, apprehensive mood, as if some misfortune were about to happen to him, or someone else, which he could in no way overcome.

CLEMATIS. He seemed oppressed by some grief or sorrow, or the shadow of some impending misfortune.

CYCLAMEN. Fretful and sad; has no desire to work; she feels a great anxiety, as if some great misfortune were impending.

GLONOINE. Feeling of impending misfortune, with sensations in the chest.

GRAPHITES. Great anxiety, in the evening, as if some misfortune had happened, with heat of the face and coldness of hands and feet.

IODUM. He fears that from every trifle some misfortune would arise.

MAGNESIA SULPHURICA. Apprehensive, tearful, very gloomy; she thought some misfortune would happen to her; especially in the morning.

NATRUM SULPHURICUM. Great fear, with dread of a misfortune.

NICCOLUM. Apprehensive and despondent, as if some misfortune were impending.

PHELLANDRIUM. Sad mood and fear the whole day, as from impending misfortune; she wept, and was prone to think upon sad subjects.

PHOSPHORUS. Anxiety, as from impending misfortune.

SULPHUR. Anxious disposition; I could not free myself from the anticipation of some great misfortune, though I had no ground for such fear, in the evening.

TABACUM. Uneasiness and anxiety in the afternoon, as if some misfortune would occur.

VERATRUM ALBUM. Anxiety as if he dreaded a misfortune, as if some evil were impending.

ZINCUM. Anxious mood, as from a misfortune.

FEAR, ghosts, of (45/I)

This fear is more common than one might suspect, though many patients are ashamed to admit it. Fear of ghosts also includes fear of spirits, of the dead, of apparitions or of anything 'from the other side'.

FEAR, high places, of (45/II)

This is also a common fear, although it is covered by only a small number of remedies. In most cases the patient will also have the symptom 'Vertigo, high places' (100/I). It should be ruled out if the fear is only of flying or of great heights. People who are genuinely scared of heights cannot stand on a first-floor balcony, and children will not climb up trees or go sledging.

FEAR, narrow place, in (46/I)

Claustrophobia is the fear or anxiety experienced in enclosed places. The classic example is a fear of lifts: some people may walk up ten flights of stairs in order to avoid having to use one. Others cannot bear doors or windows to be kept shut. (In this case one should investigate whether the symptom is not really 'Air, desire for' (1343/II) or 'Air, open, amel.' (1344/II). There are two general symptoms which are worse for confined spaces: 'Vaults, cellars, etc., agg.' (1411/I) and 'Faintness, close room, in' (1359/II). The symptom 'Anxiety, house, in' (7/I) is not always a modality of claustrophobia, though it is, for example, in the case of the remedy Tilia.

Claustrophobia may lie behind a fear of death. A female patient said she was scared of dying, and when asked why, replied without hesitation, 'Because I'm scared of being put in a coffin. I've asked my family to have me cremated when I die.' In this case the relevant symptom was clearly claustrophobia.

Materia Medica

TILIA. He cannot remain in the house on account of a sensation of apprehension and anxiety; the room seems too close, he is obliged to go into the open air, in the evening, when he feels better.

FEAR, noise, from (46/II)

This is a useful symptom during infancy, of greatest value after the age of one. Children with this symptom are afraid of the noise of car horns, engines, vacuum-cleaners and blenders. A 3-year-old girl who was sent to me was scared of popguns and balloons. Fear of noises may also indicate the symptom 'Fear, robbers, of' (47/I).

FEAR, poverty (46/II); FEAR, ruin, financial, of (47/I); FEAR, want, of (47/II)

Fear of poverty may be considered a genuine symptom in patients who suffered hardships earlier in life, provided that the fear is sufficiently marked. Businessmen and manufacturers who are always worried about the sale of their goods and live in fear of a downturn in trade belong to this rubric.

In many patients, fear of financial insecurity is accompanied by a fear of starvation, or of going hungry: 'Fear, starving, of' (47/I).

FEAR, public places, of (46/II)

This symptom, agoraphobia, is the opposite of claustrophobia. The term designates a morbid fear of crossing a wide and open space (a square or a street) on one's own, often with associated feelings of distress.

One patient told me, 'I'm scared of big empty spaces like beaches, or large squares, or the mountains. They make me feel very anxious.'

One should investigate the possible presence of agoraphobia in any patient who is scared of going out. The symptom must not however be confused with a feeling of fear or anxiety at being out of doors, when the open space is not necessarily large.

FEAR, riding, when in a carriage (47/I)

This fear is also expressed as fear of being in a car crash. One must find out whether the patient has ever actually been involved in such an accident. A curious modality, noted in many Sepia women, is a fear of being in a car driven by their husband.

FEAR, robbers, of (47/I)

Taking precautions against burglary or theft is a natural impulse in every individual. It reaches the level of a fear when one needs to obsessively check and re-check the lock on the door, look under the bed and in the wardrobe. Such people freeze on hearing the slightest suspicious noise.

FEAR, stomach, arising from (47/I); STOMACH, apprehension, in (480/I)

These two headings are in practice identical. Patients say that they have 'a feeling of fear in the stomach'. There may be no apparent cause for this symptom, or it may appear as a result of some external stimulus: bad news, pre-examination nerves, a fright, fear of thunderstorms or dogs, etc. The stimulus may also be internal – for example, the thought of something unpleasant.

One might go so far as to say that 'Apprehension in the stomach' is the repercussion of any emotion in the solar plexus. Strictly speaking, however, the symptom is present only if it fulfils one or more of the following conditions:

- There is a sensation of fear in the solar plexus, whether the stimulus is external, internal or not evident at all.
- There is a certain sensation in the epigastrium: of emptiness, weakness, trembling, constriction, a knot etc., the stimulus in this case being the fear.
- All the emotions act upon the stomach. Ideally, one of these emotions should be fear. Kent coined the term 'plexosolar' for such patients (*Lectures on Homoeopathic Materia Medica*, page 748, Mezereum).

It is often difficult to differentiate anxiety in the stomach, 'Stomach, anxiety' (476/I), from 'Stomach, apprehension, in'. As with apprehension, the anxiety may be caused by an external stimulus. This can be seen in the materia medica, in remedies such as Ferrum Metallicum: 'From slight cause, anxiety with throbbing in pit of stomach', or Lycopodium, in which this symptom is suddenly experienced when people approach him, or when he feels annoyed or angry.

Practical Examples
'Noises and emotions affect my stomach.'

'When I am in a high place, or when I feel nervous, I get butterflies in my stomach.'

'When I'm frightened or angry, or when I hear a sudden noise, I get rhythmical contractions in my stomach.' In this case (a Natrum Muriaticum woman), the symptom 'Stomach, constriction, convulsive' (483/I) was also present.

'I have a permanent feeling of anxiety in my stomach; that's the part of my body where I feel fears and frights.'

Materia Medica

CANNABIS SATIVA. He became anxious and apprehensive in the pit of the stomach, with oppression of the breath and palpitation; rising of something warm into the throat, with arrest of breathing; soon something became lodged in the trachea, with flushes of heat.

FERRUM. From slight cause, anxiety with throbbing in pit of stomach.

LYCOPODIUM. If people come near her, she is immediately attacked with anxiety at the pit of the stomach. / Great anxiety, as if in the pit of the stomach, without special thoughts. / Great apprehensiveness in the pit of the stomach, from peevishness.

MEZEREUM. Apprehensiveness in the pit of the stomach, as though expecting something disagreeable.

NATRUM MURIATICUM. Apprehensiveness, anxiety in the chest, with pressure in the pit of the stomach; worse after deep expiration.

PHOSPHORUS. When thinking of anything disagreeable, he falls into a kind of apprehension, the sensation of which is mostly in the pit of the stomach.

FEAR, thunderstorm, of (47/II)

This cannot be considered a true symptom if it developed after the patient suffered an accident caused by a storm – such as, for instance, his house being struck by lightning.

FOOLISH behaviour (48/I); SILLY (80/II); BUFFOONERY (10/I)

The materia medica does not always differentiate between symptoms of foolish behaviour and those relating to childish behaviour, but there are clear differences between the two. Foolish or clownish behaviour in children is easily observed during the consultation. These attempts to be funny or amusing often indicate that the child has low self-esteem, or it may be a means of calling for attention.

Related Symptoms
'Antics, plays' (4/I)
'Jesting, ridiculous or foolish' (60/I)
'Speech, foolish' (81/II)

Materia Medica

CARBO ANIMALIS. At times lachrymose, at times foolishly jovial.

CARBO VEGETABILIS. Sensitive, easily irritated mood, which was easily excited to foolish mirth; when laughing the muscles of the arms and hands became relaxed.

CUBEBA. Paroxysms of foolish gaiety, with great loquacity, or silent weeping, also towards evening.

CURARE. Foolish merriment, interrupted by fright and weeping. / Fits of ecstasy at night, as if caused by hearing music.

HYOSCYAMUS. Foolish actions. Comical alienation of mind; they perform ludicrous actions like monkeys.

MERCURIUS SOLUBILIS. He was foolish, played tricks, and made a fool of himself with senseless stuff; in the evening he made a fire in the stove (during the hot summer), laid swords across each other, placed lights in one corner of the room, boots in another, and all the time was fully in earnest; wherewith he was completely indifferent to warmth and cold; but his head was confused and heavy.

NUX MOSCHATA. They became foolish and delirious. / Felt foolishly happy, but could not talk; had no desire to talk. He stood still upon the street, made foolish gestures; between the attacks he sank into absence of mind, and on collecting himself everything about him seemed ludicrous. During this he looked foolish and childish, like an idiot.

PHOSPHORUS. Foolish, disconnected talking, followed by quiet delirium, with lucid intervals.

PHYSOSTIGMA. Acted foolish; said it made him crazy.

ROBINIA. Mental alienation and craziness, with furious motions or with laughter, buffoonery, jumping, and dancing.

SECALE CORNUTUM. Foolishness.

SULPHUR. When spoken to he seems absorbed, as if walking in a dream; he seems foolish; is obliged to exert himself to understand and answer correctly.

FOREBODINGS (48/II)

This symptom does not have any of its own remedies in the *Repertory*, as Kent merely refers the reader to the rubrics 'Fear' (42/II), 'Anxiety' (4/II), and 'Sadness, mental depression' (75/I). However, it deserves the attention it gets in Boenninghausen's *Characteristics and*

Repertory, where it appears as a rubric in its own right: 'Presentiments, premonitions, forebodings, etc.' (213/II).

It contains the following remedies: Aconite, Aesculus Hippocastanum, Agnus Castus, Ammonium Carbonicum, Apis Mellifica, Argentum Nitricum, Arsenicum Album, Calcarea Carbonica, Carbo Vegetabilis, Causticum, China, Elaps Corallinus, Gelsemium, Kali Carbonicum, Lachesis, Lycopodium, Medorrhinum, Naja Tripudia, Phosphorus, Plumbum, Psorinum, Sepia, Silicea, Spigelia Anthelmia, Stramonium, and Veratrum Album.

I suggest that these remedies be returned to the vacant rubric 'Forebodings' in Kent's *Repertory*.

Presentiments, premonitions and forebodings refer to a vague and disturbing feeling that something, usually bad, will happen. The divination that is typical of clairvoyance is not present.

Materia Medica

CALCAREA CARBONICA. Despairing mood, with dread of disease and suffering, with foreboding of sad events.

KALI CARBONICUM. He has anxious presentiments, in the evening. / Sad presentiments of the future. / At night after lying down, sad forebodings overtake him, on account of which he is unable to sleep.

NABALUS. Vague and sinister presentiments, in the mornings.

NATRUM PHOSPHORICUM. Misgivings.

PHOSPHORUS. Filled with gloomy forebodings.

PSORINUM. Anxiety, full of forebodings, very restless, with trembling of the hands.

SEPIA. Dark forebodings about his disease in regard to the future.

STILLINGIA SYLVATICA. Depression of spirits (eleventh day), and gloomy forebodings, low spirits.

FORSAKEN feeling (49/I); LONELINESS (63/I)

A close reading of Hahnemann's *Materia Medica Pura* shows that this symptom should be taken to mean the following:
- The feeling of being alone, forsaken.
- The feeling that he is not loved, that he has lost his friends (modalities of Aurum, Hura and other remedies).
- A fear of loneliness, 'of being left on one's own in life', expressed in a fear of the death of those closest to him. (This is the traditional clinical modality, frequently found in Calcarea Carbonica patients.)

Practical Examples

'I'm scared of not being loved, of being abandoned by the people I love, by my girlfriend, my father, and my brother and sister. I feel as though they're deserting me, and it frightens me.' (19-year-old man.)

'I crave affection, I need it, I'm terrified of being left. When I was small I used to complain that my mother loved my brothers and sisters more than me, and when I was seven I packed up my teddy bear and wanted to run away from home, I told my father and mother that they didn't love me.' (35-year-old woman)

(A 5-year-old girl): 'She gets terribly upset' (explained her mother) 'when the others won't play with her at the nursery school. The other day she cried bitterly when her little cousin told her that she didn't love her any more. She'll do anything her friends tell her for fear of losing them.'

(Patricia, aged 23): 'As a child I was very affectionate. If someone didn't love me I felt it was the end of the world. My whole life revolved around whether my parents loved me or not. If they lost their temper with me, I thought that they didn't love me. I used to wonder why Daddy wasn't affectionate all the time.'

All four of these patients were Pulsatilla. Sometimes women express this symptom when they complain that their families don't pay attention to them or that their relatives never come and visit them.

Materia Medica

AURUM. He is dejected and seeks solitude. He imagines he has lost the affection of his friends; this makes him sad, even to tears.

CALCAREA CARBONICA. Loneliness is very oppressive, with coldness of the face, hands and feet.

CARBO ANIMALIS. Extremely melancholy mood, with feeling of being abandoned. Discouraged and sad; everything seems so sad and lonely that she desires to weep.

HURA BRASILIENSIS. She fancies she is left alone in the world and is lost.

KALI BROMATUM. She had the erroneous idea that she was deserted by all her friends, and as a consequence passed all her waking moments, which were not many, in tears.

KALI CARBONICUM. Sad, lonely; she seeks society in order to enliven herself.

KEROSOLENUM. As you breathe the vapour you seem to float away into a wavy maze, with a sense of complete loneliness; there appears to be but one object in the universe, and that object is yourself; on recovery the first thing seen is deemed the only thing existing in the universe; it takes some little time to regain all the faculties.

LAMIUM. Weeping mood; she wept as if she had been abandoned.

NATRUM CARBONICUM. She does not know what to do, on account of apprehensiveness and ennui. Thinks she is quite lonely and forsaken, all day.

PLATINUM. It seems to her as if she does not belong in her own family; after a short absence everything seems entirely changed. She thinks she is left wholly to herself, and stands alone in the world. Very restless disposition, so that she cannot remain anywhere; sad, so that the most joyful things distress her; thinks she has no place in the world, life is wearisome; has a great dread of death, which she believes to be near at hand.

PULSATILLA. It seems so quiet in her head and everything feels so empty that she seems alone in the house and in the world; she will speak to no one, just as if her surroundings did not exist, and she pays attention to no one.

RHUS TOXICODENDRON. Melancholy, ill-humour and anxiety, as if a misfortune would happen, or as if she were alone and all about her were dead and still, or as if she had been forsaken by a near friend; worse in the house, relieved by walking in the open air.

FRIVOLOUS (50/I)

The frivolous person is vacuous and superficial.

Rakish and dissolute, this sensualist surrenders to every whim. He is devoted to casual relationships, drunkeness, debauchery, fine cigarettes, wild parties and pornographic films. His sole ideal is the pleasure of empty distraction. He achieves nothing important or substantial.

FROWN, disposed to (50/I)

Frowning may be readily observed in a patient. This manner of expressing displeasure, deep thought, irritation, and so on, is an interesting and useful symptom.

Care must be taken to distinguish it from 'Face, wrinkled, forehead' (396/II). The latter is a sign of age, or may accompany migraines, respiratory or cerebral conditions.

GRIEF, ailments, from (51/I)

This generally applies to patients in whom various ailments have been brought on by the grief of losing a loved one. In identifying the symptom, one must ascertain in each case whether the feeling was genuinely one of grief, and not of fear, loss of support, guilt, etc.

It is also found in those who fall ill when a member of the family goes away: a 6-year-old boy suffered character changes, depression and severe attacks of asthma whenever his father was away on business.

Practical Examples

'I've been poorly since my father died two years ago. I'm always depressed and I suffer from headaches, giddy spells and nausea.'

'I've had vitiligo and asthma for fourteen years, since my father died. I think of him and talk about him with my children as though he were still alive.' (*Cries*) The symptom 'Inconsolable' (54/I) also applied to this patient.

GRIEF, silent (51/I)

This simply refers to those who do not share their grief with anyone. It is generally to be found in reserved people (see 'Reserved' (72/I)).

Practical Examples

'I am a very quiet person. I don't tell anyone about my problems, not even my mother, because I don't want to trouble them.'

'I never complain or ask for sympathy. I'm very resigned – no one knows I'm sad because I keep it to myself.'

'My husband died twelve years ago. My children don't know that I'm sad and cry every day. I've always concealed it. You're the first person I've told, Doctor.'

Materia Medica

NUX VOMICA. Silent grief and sadness.

HAUGHTY (51/II); ARROGANCE (9/I); PRIDE (69/II); IMPERIOUS (54/I)

'Haughty' is closely related to the symptoms 'Egotism' (39/I) and 'Contemptuous' (16/I). Kent cross-references 'Arrogance', 'Pride' and 'Imperious' to it. The proud person is characterised by a great feeling of his own worth. He is pleased with himself.

The haughty person may be recognised as much by what he tells you as by his arrogant attitude and bearing. He is the great braggart who makes a show of being more than he really is. In his vanity he thinks that he is better than everyone else. He wants to be famous and respected. He is the pompous pedant who makes a show of his erudition.

A haughty and arrogant attitude usually conceals a deep sense of inferiority.

Related Symptoms
'Conceit' (Paschero: Lachesis, Nux Vomica, Platinum, Veratrum Album)
'Delusions, humility and lowness of others, while he is great' (27/II)
'Delusions, inferior, on entering house, after a walk, people seem mentally and physically' (28/I)
'Delusions, superiority' (33/I)
'Presumptuous' (69/II)

Related Symptom in the Synthetic Repertory
'Vanity' (column 1055)

Practical Examples
(A woman, of her husband): 'His worst fault is that he thinks he knows everything – he's a walking encyclopaedia.'
'As a boy I was very self-important. I was always top of the class, and held everyone else in contempt, and for that reason I didn't have many friends. I wanted to be the best at everything, I was more than a little arrogant and I tried to impose my views on everyone.'

Materia Medica
HAMAMELIS. Feeling that she ought to be reverenced by all around her and have great respect paid to her opinions.
PLATINUM. Arrogant, proud feeling.
ROBINIA. Anxiety to seek honours; excessive pride; he considers himself better than an emperor.

HEEDLESS (51/II); CARELESS (10/I)

This is a relatively important symptom, generally associated with 'Chaotic' (10/II). The heedless person is sometimes scatter-brained or inattentive, and always negligent.

Practical Examples
'David (aged nine) is very careless. He opens drawers and then forgets to close them. When he gets out of the car he leaves the door open.'
'Samantha (eleven) is careless. She has already lost three watches – she loses everything.'
'When William goes to school forgets to take half the things he needs. Yesterday he lost a textbook, and he's gone through goodness knows how many coats. He even loses things he cares about, like his football.'

HELPLESSNESS, feeling of (51/II)

There have been problems with the definition of this symptom. Some homoeopaths take it to mean 'feels powerless, unable to do anything', others 'feels as though he has been deserted', while for a third party it suggests the sense of being unprotected and defenceless. In fact, these are all just different ways in which patients express the same symptom.

It should not be confused with 'Forsaken feeling' (49/II), which signifies a lack of support and care when one cannot look after oneself.

Practical Examples
(A 32-year-old woman): 'I couldn't do without support from someone else'. (On another occasion) 'When I go to stay with my mother and father I sleep well because I feel safe.' (On a third occasion) 'My husband died of a heart attack and now I have so many responsibilities. I can't cope, I feel so helpless and alone.'
'I feel vulnerable and unprotected. I need someone to lean on.'
(A hospital doctor): 'My lack of self-confidence began when I was fourteen, when my mother died. I felt helpless, I had no support. Now I get upset whenever I feel powerless to help my patients.'

Materia Medica
ETHER. His sensations were so dreadful that he would rather undergo any amount of pain than submit to the same again, which he could compare only to a state of utter helplessness and impending dissolution.

JASMINUM. Weak and almost helpless for a few days.
KALI BROMATUM. Dull, depressed, irregular in his gait, in the morning; in the afternoon completely helpless.
LYCOPODIUM. The thoughts seem to stand still; the mind is helpless and as if dazed, like a confusion, without obscuration of mind.
TAXUS. State of profound stupor and helplessness.

HOME, desires to leave (51/II)

This symptom is as curious as it is useful. Found especially in children, who threaten to leave home after being scolded, smacked or ignored in some way. Of course the threat is never actually carried out. I have observed this behaviour in Veratrum Album patients.

Practical Examples
(A mother said of her 5-year-old daughter): 'When she gets annoyed she says she will leave us and leave home.'
'She's always saying that she'll pack her things up and leave home because we don't love her any more.' (4-year-old girl)
'On several occasions after I had given Laura a telling-off she packed up her clothes and toys and said she was going to her aunt's.'

HOMESICKNESS (51/II)

Homesickness is an ailment brought on by absence from one's home, family or friends. It is the distressing memory of something that has been lost. One can see it in elderly immigrants in whom the passing of time has not effaced a longing for their native land.

Practical Examples
'It's three years since I retired from my job as a nurse at the hospital. Every time I go past the hospital gates I burst into tears, I miss it so much. Another thing that grieves me is that one of my daughters got married and moved to Italy. I miss her all the time.'
(A 45-year-old woman): 'I spend all my time thinking about how happy my childhood was. Whenever I hear a tango I burst into tears. I'm like a ninety-year-old, all I have is my memories.'
'When we moved house, it was a great shock to my son. He's always asking me if we can go back to see the place where we used to live.'

Homesickness

(A young man of twenty): 'I feel overwhelmed by my memories. I'd like to be back at school, I miss my friends.'

Materia Medica

CARBO ANIMALIS. In the morning, he felt abandoned and homesick.

CARLSBAD. Mood very much depressed, like an excessive homesickness; in the end weeps violently.

CENTAUREA TAGANA. Homesickness.

CLEMATIS. Irritable, angry, fretful, avoiding everyone, shunning his usually agreeable occupations, dreading to be alone, tired of living, full of thoughts of death, with fear that it would be speedy; longing, however, for the repose of death; this mood was soon followed by apprehension, weeping, and homesickness, at last outbreak of tears, with most violent trembling of the whole body and weeping for half an hour until he was completely exhausted and compelled to rest.

EUPATORIUM PURPUREUM. Homesick, though occupying her own home and surrounded by her own family.

HELLEBORUS. Homesickness.

HIPPOMANES. Homesick in the evening.

HYOSCYAMUS. Remembrance of long-past events. Curative action? (Hahnemann.)

MAGNESIA MURIATICA. Was apprehensive, despondent and lonesome; was homesick and wept.

MERCURIUS SOLUBILIS. Longing for home.

NITRIC ACIDUM. Homesickness.

PLANTAGO. Feeling great desire to be at home when abroad.

PULSATILLA NUTTALLIANA. Great depression of spirits, in the afternoon; a kind of homesickness, with despondency.

SACCHARUM ALBUM. Indifference, as from homesickness.

SENECIO. Homesickness.

SILICEA. Longing for home.

HOPEFUL (52/I)

'Hopeful' should be combined with 'Optimistic' (*Synthetic Repertory*, column 792) because they are difficult to tell apart in practice.

These people always remain calm in the most difficult situations, confident that everything will turn out for the best. They are generally cheerful people with an excessively rosy view of the future. Their catch-phrases are 'Everything will turn out right' and 'Don't worry'.

Materia Medica

FERRUM MAGNETICUM. Hopeful with hilarity and confidence in the future.

HYDRASTIS. Unusual cheerfulness and hopefulness, several days.

KALI CARBONICUM. Alternating mood; at one time good and quiet, at another excited and angry at trifles; frequently hopeful, frequently despondent.

RAPHANUS. Capricious mania, stupefaction, sadness and tears, alternating with hopefulness; she fears she will become a burden to everyone.

HOPELESS (52/I)

This symptom should likewise be combined with 'Pessimistic' (*Synthetic Repertory*, column 794).

The hopeless person or pessimist suffers from a feeling of sadness and a lack of self-confidence. Life, according to him, is beset with difficulties and the future is always associated with problems. He sees the worst side of everything and his catchphrase is 'There's nothing to be done', for he believes all endeavours to be useless. A patient said, 'I have no hope or faith, I doubt everything, I'm fatalistic, I don't think that one can do anything to change the course of events.' Another patient told me, 'I live in a state of anguish and despair, as though my whole world was about to collapse. I feel I don't have a future.'

Kent's *Repertory* lists no remedies under 'Hopeless' and the reader is referred to 'Despair' (35/II), which has two important modalities: 'Despair, recovery' (36/I) and 'Despair, religious (of salvation, etc.)' (36/I).

Note also two distinct but closely-related symptoms: 'Doubtful, recovery, of' (37/I), and 'Doubtful, soul's welfare, of' (37/I).

Materia Medica

CARBO ANIMALIS. Hopelessness.

FERRUM PHOSPHORICUM. Early in the evening loss of courage and hope; better since sleeping.

GADUS MORRHUA. Deep melancholy, paroxysms of hopelessness, for forty-eight hours, during which the desire for death is hardly controlled. The intellectual faculties are torpid.

GRAPHITES. Grief about the slightest ocurrences, even to despair.

MORPHINUM. Some patients sit in mute despair, casting about for some opportunity to free themselves from their suffering.

NATRUM CARBONICUM. Very fretful and discontented with the whole world; he constantly felt as though he could beat himself, his whole life angered him, and he preferred to have no existence at all; he was solicitous about the future, and inclined to despair, all day.

NATRUM MURIATICUM. Attacks of complete hopelessness and internal despair, that deprived him of all power. / Although a well-educated and intelligent woman, her mind seemed hopeless and confused.

NITRICUM ACIDUM. Boundless despair.

OPIUM. Hopeless, morose mood, fretfulness.

PSORINUM. Very melancholy and despairing; he wishes to die in spite of his good luck.

SECALE CORNUTUM. Loathing of life; despair.

THUJA. Mood very unhappy, despairing. / Constant great despair changes at last to complete indifference. / Increasing despair which allows rest nowhere, seemed to be intolerable day and night.

WIESBADEN. Impatient and depressed, without hope.

HORRIBLE things, sad stories, affect her profoundly (52/I)

This symptom is summed up by the word 'impressionable'. It should not be confused with the symptom 'Sympathetic' (86/I). An impressionable patient experiences a sudden and profound feeling of anxiety at the sight of scenes which may sometimes be sad, but are usually violent and bloody.

As with other symptoms, one must take into account both the cause and the nature of the patient's reaction. If the patient says that the sight of an injured person would deeply affect him, but would not prevent him from giving assistance, then this particular symptom is not present.

People who are truly impressionable feel horrified. They are powerless to help and can even faint. Such children cry when they see monsters on television or at the cinema; adults get upset when they see scenes of violence. The sight of blood, a street fight, an accident, death, even injections, operations or the merest whiff of hospital disinfectant is enough to scare the wits out of them.

Related Symptoms
'Anxiety, cruelties, after hearing of' (6/I)
'Excitement, horrible things, after hearing' (40/II)
'Fear, cruelties, report of, excite' (43/II)

'Sensitive, cruelties, when hearing of' (78/II)
'Talking, unpleasant things, of, agg.' (87/I)

Related Symptoms in the Synthetic Repertory
'Anguish, horrible things, after hearing' (column 44)
'Fear, see wounds, to' (column 521)
'Impressionable' (column 606)

Practical Examples
'The slightest cut or graze makes me feel very anxious, and then my blood pressure goes down. Once I got terribly upset when I saw a shop assistant fall off his stepladder.'
'The smell of a hospital is enough to make me faint. I once fainted when I had an injection.'
'I can't bear to watch boxing or war films. I feel squeamish whenever I see an invalid or a funeral cortege.'
'I once fainted when I went to the dentist's with my wife.'
'I don't watch violent or grisly programmes on television. In fact I don't even watch the news.'

Materia Medica
CICUTA VIROSA. Anxiety, he is excessively affected by sad stories.
NATRUM CARBONICUM. Every event makes a strong impression upon her; a wavy trembling in the nerves, with a sensation of faintness.

HURRY (52/I)

The hurried person is easy to identify. He will often reveal himself by the way he introduces himself to you, by his attitude and speech. These people do everything in great haste. They sometimes talk and act so hurriedly that other people may feel quite crushed in their presence. They may even undertake several tasks at the same time.

One should take care to establish that there is no logical reason for the symptom; some patients do everything rapidly simply because they are pressed for time and have much to do.

When the patient speaks quickly, the appropriate symptom is 'Speech, hasty' (81/II). If he shows haste in two or more kinds of action then the general symptom applies. The symptom 'Hurry, eating, while' (52/I) is quite common – a result of the pressures of daily life – and should thus be treated with caution.

Practical Examples
'Even if I've got lots of time I still hurry.'
'I'm a walking disaster area. I do everything in a hurry, twenty things at the same time.'
'I run even if I'm in good time.'
'In a hurry, I want to do everything quickly, I hurry so much that I start to bump into things, then I feel sorry for myself, wring my hands, trip up over things.'

IMPATIENCE (53/II)

In many patients, this symptom is accompanied by feelings of haste and restlessness.

The *Encyclopaedia of Pure Materia Medica* shows that in almost every instance where 'Impatience' occurs in a prover, it is almost always accompanied by irritability. Indeed, in the case of Zincum, it was thought necessary to explain that the prover was 'very impatient, but not, however, irritable'.

The patient grumbles, is intolerant, upset by setbacks. He finds it impossible to wait, no matter for whom or what, becoming uneasy and irritable to such a degree that he needs to flee the situation at whatever cost or effort this may involve. He will walk up ten flights of stairs rather than wait for the lift; faced by a traffic jam he will turn off into side streets that he doesn't know; rather than wait his turn after a couple of patients in the waiting room he will make another appointment, provided that he will then be seen first.

On one occasion a patient came in to my surgery and exclaimed angrily, 'This is an insult, I'm a psychologist and I have patients to see too – my time is every bit as valuable as yours . . .' I realised that this was a case of wounded pride rather than impatience, and prescribed Lycopodium.

Practical Examples
'I sometimes walk ten blocks rather than wait for the bus.'
'I don't have patience for anything; I'll walk up the stairs rather than wait for a lift, or make a huge detour to avoid the traffic lights.'
'I don't wait for anything – I can't bear to queue at the petrol station.'
'I'm very impatient. When people talk to me, I ask them to get to the point of what they are saying. I start a book and skip whole chapters in order to get to the end.'

IMPERTINENCE (54/I)

Impertinence and insolence are synonyms, which is why in the *Repertory* we find the same remedies under both headings. 'Insolent' actually has some additional remedies, and is the one that should be referred to.

IMPETUOUS (54/I)

This symptom does not limit itself to fits of anger, but extends beyond the aggressive instincts so that every single act and movement is performed precipitately, unexpectedly and with a force that is almost violent. The replies of an impetuous person are characteristically rapid and intense.

Materia Medica

FERRUM PHOSPHORICUM. Evening, impetuous feeling, yet obstacles cause annoyance and hesitation, and trifles seem like mountains, still intolerant of hindrance and annoyance.

LAUROCERASUS. Hasty, impetuous.

SULPHUR. Morose and impetuous.

IMPULSIVE (54/I)

This symptom is closely related to 'Impetuous' (54/I). The difference between them is that the impulsive person never thinks before he acts; he has no concept of intention or deliberation. A momentary impression causes him to react suddenly, either verbally or physically. He only realizes the implications of his actions afterwards. Many patients who report the symptom regret this embarrassing and potentially dangerous lack of self-control.

Practical Examples

'I'm impulsive, I don't put up with things, I'm not very tactful.'
'I act without thinking.'
'I'm very impulsive, I don't think about what I'm saying, I say something and then regret it.'
'I'm what you might call explosive, extremely impulsive. I react very rashly and then regret it afterwards. A few days ago one of my

employees made some slight error and I violently insulted him for it. Unfortunately some clients were looking on and they were shocked by my outburst. Once, during an argument with my wife, I put my fist through a door, and another time I threw the television set on the floor.'
'As a child I used to react violently, I never stopped to think.'
'I'm impulsive, I react violently, explosively. In the heat of the moment I kick the furniture and break things. I was very violent with my first wife. I used to beat her – I didn't know what I was doing.'
'I'm very explosive and impulsive; I say things without thinking and then regret it bitterly.'
'I can't stop myself from saying hurtful things to people.'
'I can't control myself.'

Materia Medica
ARSENICUM ALBUM. Feeling of impulsiveness.
GINSENG. Mind generally calm; still there are impatient impulses and fear of accidents, with, at times, disposition to weep, or to be anxious about the future.

INCONSOLABLE (54/I)

The inconsolable person is by definition always sad. Grief-stricken, he cannot take his mind off the catastrophe that has befallen him. Usually this is the death of a loved one, but it could also be the theft of something precious, or the loss of his house in a fire. What was taken from him cannot be restored, and therein lies his misfortune. Neither the passage of time, nor words of reason or religious consolation, bring any relief.

In cases of bereavement, the mourning process is held up. Coming to terms with a death is an arduous task which the inconsolable person tries to put off, clinging to the notion that the deceased is still alive. Other kinds of loss may actually be wholly imaginary. In my experience, one or more of the following features are often present:
- The prior existence of a strong emotional bond with the loved one.
- Symptoms of remorse when there was an element of conflict in the relationship with the deceased. There is a feeling of guilt if the patient sees the death as something that was wished for. In this case, the symptom 'Anxiety, conscience, of', is also present.
- The love was not experienced on a mature level, and the loved one was merely a provider of necessities.

Though the last two cases are self-explanatory, the symptom must be taken at face value if there is a real and lasting sense of grief and misfortune.

Practical Examples
'My mother has been dead these last seventeen years and I still can't accept the fact. I talk about her in the present tense as though she were still alive.' (57-year-old woman)
'I fell ill when my mother died eighteen years ago. I never got over it, I felt as though I had lost half of myself. I couldn't face life without her because she always helped me with all my problems.' (The symptom 'Grief, ailments, from' (51/I) was also present in this case.)
'I was widowed twenty years ago and still haven't come to terms with it. He's always on my mind, I keep thinking that he'll come back to me.'
'Daddy died seven years ago. It was a terrible shock. I still talk to him and write him letters.' (25-year-old woman)
'My brother was killed in an accident, and I hid myself away and cried for a year. Nothing could console me.' (42-year-old woman)

Materia Medica
ACONITUM. Inconsolable anxiety and piteous howlings, with complaints and reproaches about trifles.
CHINA. Inconsolable.
NATRUM CARBONICUM. Ill-humour, discontented and almost inconsolable.
NUX VOMICA. Extremely solicitous and inconsolable; breaks out into loud weeping, with complaints and reproaches that at times change to constant groaning, with very red, hot cheeks, without thirst.
PHOSPHORUS. Inconsolable grief, with weeping and crying; in the morning.
PLATINUM. She sits alone, sad and morose, without talking, she cannot keep awake; followed by inconsolable weeping, especially when spoken to.
STRAMONIUM. She is all the time inconsolable; much affected by trifles; makes much fuss about trifles; disposed to weep, and sometimes also very easily vexed.
VERATRUM ALBUM. She is inconsolable over a fancied misfortune, runs about the room howling and screaming, looking upon the ground, or sits brooding in the corner, wailing and weeping in an inconsolable manner; worse in the evening, sleeps only till 2 o'clock.

INCONSTANCY (54/I)

Inconstant people are always changing their plans, objectives and jobs. They start something with great enthusiasm but the novelty does not last for long, for they soon lose interest and abandon it. Then at once they take up with something else, and so it goes on.

Their lives are a catalogue of careers cut short, of courses dropped, of girlfriends that they left because they got bored with them, of a variety of different doctors, none of whom could come up with quick results. Everything they do bears the seal of their inconstancy.

Related Symptoms
'Persists in nothing' (69/II)
'Undertakes many things, perseveres in nothing' (91/I)

A symptom frequently associated with 'Inconstancy' is 'Mood, changeable, variable, etc.' (68/I). This may be expressed as a fluctuation between two opposing poles, such as joy and sadness, or as movement through widely differing states of mind – irritability, happiness, anxiety, apathy, activity, excitement, dejection, etc. These people say that they are unstable or prone to swings in mood. They may be impressionable and affected by the slightest things.

INDIFFERENCE (54/II)

Although indifference is common in cases of melancholy, it is most useful when the modalities are analysed. The most common and characteristic modalities are 'Indifference, everything, to' and 'Indifference, pleasure, to'.

INDIFFERENCE, everything, to (55/I)

These are truly apathetic people, who have lost interest in even those things that used to interest them. They are cold, joyless, humourless, say little and hardly smile.

Practical Examples
'Nothing interests me, I have no desire to do anything, I no longer enjoy cooking. I hate work of all kinds. I don't often feel like talking.'

'I have no enthusiasm for anything, everything seems quite monotonous, I just don't see the point.' 'All I want to do is to stay in bed. I don't watch TV, I don't read the paper, nothing interests me. I don't have a sex life, my wife can't stand me any more. I don't even feel like going to visit my factory.'

Materia Medica

ARNICA. Indifference to everything.

BOVISTA. In company she was lively; alone, sad, depressed, and not interested in anything.

CANNABIS SATIVA. Nothing pleases him; he is indifferent to everything.

CAPSICUM. Indifferent to everything.

CARBO VEGETABILIS. Indifferent, not interested in anything. / He heard everything without feeling pleasantly or unpleasantly about it, and without thinking of it. / Music, of which he is fond, does not interest him the whole day.

CHAMOMILLA. Want of attention, careless; external objects make no impression upon him; he is indifferent to everything.

CICUTA VIROSA. He was indifferent to everything, and began to doubt whether he was really in the condition in which he found himself.

CINA. Indifference; neither agreeable nor disagreeable things make the slightest impression upon him.

CROCUS. Indifference to everything.

CROTALUS HORRIDUS. Depression, and indifference to everything.

CUBEBA. Fits of dejection, apathy, insensibility; is indifferent to everything.

CURARE. Indifference to everything going on about him.

DIGITALIS. Very indifferent to everything, for several days.

FERRUM. Ill humour; disinclined for everything; indifferent even to subjects in which he usually took an active interest; joyfulness was impossible.

IGNATIA. Indifferent to everything; he seemed to live without his usual good humour.

KALI CARBONICUM. Disinclined to everything, and indifferent.

LEPIDIUM. Want of ideas; inability to think; with indifference to everything.

MERCURIUS SOLUBILIS. Cared for nothing, and was indifferent to everything. / He was indifferent; had no desire to eat and yet, when he ate, relished his food and took as much as usual.

MEZEREUM. Indifferent to everything; he could scarcely compel himself to note the symptoms beyond brief annotations (as in sea-sickness).

NUX MOSCHATA. Absence of mind, cannot think; great indifference to everything; scalp very much stretched, he laid down at noon.

PHOSPHORUS. Great indifference to everything.

SECALE CORNUTUM. Indifference to everything.

SEPIA. Great indifference towards everything; no proper sense of life.

STAPHYSAGRIA. Mind phlegmatic, depressed, sad, apathetic, indifferent to everything, without peevishness or without being weak.

INDIFFERENCE, loved ones, to (55/I)

Indifference to one's loved ones, or emotional indifference, is a symptom that belongs to the deepest level of the human psyche – what Kent called the level of the will. When it is disturbed, it gives rise to symptoms such as hate, suicide, aversion to and hatred of one's family.

Emotional indifference is found in the *Repertory* under the following headings:

'Indifference, her children, to' (55/I)

'Indifference, loved ones, to' (55/I)

'Indifference, relations, to' (55/I)

It is interesting to note that some remedies are common to both the 'Indifference' and 'Aversion' rubrics. For example, 'Indifference, relations, to' and 'Aversion, members of family, to' (9/I) share the following remedies: Fluoricum Acidum, Natrum Carbonicum and Sepia.

Practical Examples

'I don't have any patience with my children. My husband is very good, my children are adorable, but I can't appreciate them.'

'I'm always watching over my children, I'm overprotective of them, and yet I get cross when they touch me or pester me. I left the family for a while ten years ago because I felt suffocated by the kids.'

Materia Medica

HELLEBORUS NIGER. Happy carelessness about everything; feels indifferent to family.

LYCOPODIUM. She feeds from her own children.

PHOSPHORUS. Indifferent to her child, of whom she was usually fond.

SEPIA. Forgot that she had her children to dress and provide for until nearly 10 o'clock.

INDIFFERENCE, others, toward (55/I)

This heading, along with that of 'Indifference, welfare of others, to' (55/II) are, in the Sulphur patient, modalities of his egoism. At his first consultation, a 32-year-old bachelor told me, 'I feel emotionally paralysed, indifferent to other people.' I prescribed Sulphur, and ten months later he was able to say, 'I've noticed that I'm less selfish, I think about other people more. I'm more altruistic.'

INDIFFERENCE, personal appearance (55/I)

In the *Repertory*, only Sulphur has this symptom, but it is in the third grade. It may be observed directly; such patients are always untidy when they come to see you, and their shoes are never clean. The wife of one patient said, 'He couldn't care less about his appearance – he would be quite happy to go around in the same clothes for a whole month.'

INDIFFERENCE, pleasure, to (55/I)

Indifference to pleasure is frequently associated with indifference to everything. This kind of person cannot enjoy anything.

Practical Examples
'I used to be able to take pleasure even in little things, but I've lost my zest for life. If I won a million dollars I wouldn't feel happy. I used to enjoy lots of things; now I just feel sorry for people.'
'Nothing arouses my interest or enthusiasm, I can't enjoy things. I don't have any kind of ambition. It wouldn't even interest me to go on holiday to some exotic place.'

Materia Medica
COCCULUS. He has no desire, and takes pleasure in nothing.
IPECACUANHA. Takes no delight in anything; nothing pleases him.
KALI CARBONICUM. Very peevish, has no joy in anything.
MEZEREUM. Hypochondriacal and despondent; takes no pleasure in anything; everything seems to him dead, and nothing makes a vivid impression upon his mind.
PRUNUS SPINOSA. Joyless mood, satisfaction with nothing.

SARSAPARILLA. Has aversion for everything; nothing gives her pleasure; only in the forenoon.

SULPHUR. She takes pleasure in nothing.

INDIGNATION (55/II)

The modality 'Indignation, bad effects following' (55/II) is often confused with 'Mortification, ailments after' (68/II), because in both cases the patient suffers as a result of what he feels is an insult to his person. While both symptoms may be present at the same time, the difference lies in the fact that in 'Indignation' a feeling of anger is always present.

Those who are easily roused to indignation have an exaggerated sense of honour, honesty and justice. A key phrase is, 'I hate any kind of injustice'. Such patients will react angrily at any sign of unmerited privilege; queue-jumpers arouse their contempt, for they feel strongly that everyone must wait their turn.

Related Symptoms
'Anger, ailments after, with indignation' (2/II)
'Honour, effects of wounded' (52/I)

The former symptom should be combined with the heading 'Indignation', which will then include Lycopodium, Mercurius Vivus and Natrum Muriaticum. These constitutional types are often indignant.

Related Symptom in the Synthetic Repertory
'Injustice, cannot support' (column 633)

Practical Examples
'The professor's post wasn't allocated on the basis of open competition. I intend to register a complaint with the Faculty, even if it costs me my career. It makes me so angry.'
'I hate deception; the Government should all be strung up.'
'Injustices sicken me; I have no respect for authority.'
'I'm definitely not one to turn the other cheek when I see people being treated unfairly. I shall speak to the boss on behalf of everyone who has been overlooked. I'll take his cronies down a peg or two – they really make me sick.'
'I'm on a short fuse when it comes to injustice – it makes me feel angry and bitter. That's why I chose to work for the social services.'

'The company for whom I had worked for seventeen years was taken over; I was third in charge and they made me redundant. I was terribly indignant and I've been poorly since then. My nerves are bad, I'm intolerant, I often raise my voice. I've become a different person.'
'It really needles me when someone double-parks or hogs the fast lane. I get annoyed when people show no respect for the rights of others. One thing I really can't stand is waiting to be served in a shop and someone coming in and asking for this or that without waiting his turn.'

Materia Medica

ARSENICUM. Indignation in the morning when in bed; pushes the pillows about indignantly, uncovers himself, sees no one, and does not want to be spoken to. / Indignation, alternating with mildness; in her indignation she looks at nobody, and does not want to hear anything; she also cries.

CALCAREA PHOSPHORICA. Unpleasant news makes him beside himself, sweat breaks out; inclined to indignation and anger.

CHINA. Fretful and irresolute; she is unable to accomplish her aim, and consequently is indignant.

FERRUM PHOSPHORICUM. Indignation for causes followed by oppression of left chest and stomach.

 **INDOLENCE, aversion to work (55/II);
AMBITION, loss of (1/II)**

Indolence must be differentiated from asthenia, or physiological inactivity, when there is a physical explanation for the symptom.

The truly lazy person does not lack energy. Lazy children play and run and jump just as much as their friends, but when it comes to studying, helping with the housework or running an errand, they simply don't have the strength to do it. They hoard their energy and use it only for those few things that really interest them.

These people have no ambition. They are known by a host of popular names: lazybones, good-for-nothing, sluggard, layabout, etc. (See 'Business, averse to' (10/I).)

Practical Examples

'Veronica won't do things she doesn't like. She spends hours cooking because she loves it, but I just can't make her do her homework or

have a bath. She likes being with her friend but she won't make the effort to phone her or go round and see her.'
'Natalia is completely lazy. She likes to sit back in an armchair, put her feet up and watch television. Whenever she wants something she asks one of us to get it for her.'
'She doesn't do as well as she could at school because she's lazy – she prefers to take it easy. When she was younger she had a strong aversion to anything that involved physical exercise.'

Related Symptoms in the Synthetic Repertory
'Ambition, loss of' (column 23)
'Idleness' (column 597). This symptom is covered in Kent's *Repertory* by the rubric 'Indolence' (55/II), taken from T. F. Allen's *Encyclopaedia of Pure Materia Medica*.

Materia Medica
ALOE. Great laziness in the middle of the day. Much exhaustion and laziness.

BORAX. He idles through the afternoon, does not really get at his work; changes from one business to another, from one room to another; does not keep at one business. / Disinclined to work; he does only what he is obliged to as if by force.

BROMIUM. He becomes averse to his business, it seems as though he must relinquish it.

BUFO. Lazy and discouraged.

CANTHARIS. Very morose, lazy, sleepy, melancholy, peevish.

CAUSTICUM. Very fretful and indolent.

CHINA. No desire for work; he is inactive.

CINA. Complete disinclination for work.

COCA. Not in humour to study or read journals; lazy and sleepy.

COCCULUS. No desire to work.

ELAPS. Aversion to work.

NATRUM CARBONICUM. Mood sluggish, phlegmatic, indolent. / Dislike for business; he goes about idly, but when once at work, it goes on as usual.

PAULLINIA PINNATA. Lazy and disinclined to work.

PHYSOSTIGMA. Perfect impossibility to concentrate my mind or to translate a single line (fourth day); perfect disinclination to any mental work; laziness and apathy reign supreme.

ROBINIA. Laziness and apathy, with desire to stay in bed all the time.

SPONGIA. Fretful and lazy; wished to rest and was little inclined to talk.

INDUSTRIOUS (56/I); WORK, mania to (95/II);
ACTIVITY, desires (1/II)

Industriousness – a devotion to hard work – is often of course an entirely normal characteristic.

This is confirmed by the materia medica, where remedies such as China, Digitalis and Ledum show great activity and industriousness in their curative symptoms. The value of the symptom naturally increases the more marked it is; some people have a real mania for work. The industrious person, in contrast to the one who is better for being occupied (see 'Occupation, amel.' (69/I)), does things that are always productive and can continue to enjoy leisure periods.

Materia Medica

CHINA. Desire for work, to read, to write, to reflect; a general, remarkable activity and industriousness (curative action).

DIGITALIS. Inclination for mental labour and all kinds of business (curative action).

IGNATIA. Very busy mood; he does now this, now that, in a restless way.

INDIGO. Great desire to work.

LACHESIS. He wishes to do a great deal; begins many things. / Need of being very busy, without the slightest perseverance. / He sits up late at night at mental work, with great activity. / He is impelled to productive work in the evening, although he had been much fatigued during the day; he sits all night, without the slightest sleepiness or exhaustion; writes with the greatest freedom and increased vigour about everything that he knows; new things constantly throng in his mind; also next day, after very little sleep, he is just as excited; it only gradually diminishes without subsequent reaction of mind; on repeated provings.

LEDUM. Joyous mood, with desire for activity and contentment with himself (curative action). (Hahnemann)

LYCOPODIUM. Excited, busy mood in the evening, without perseverance, changing from one subject to another, with difficulty in fixing the thoughts, and greater difficulty in accomplishing anything; while reading fell asleep.

OPIUM. Felt an intense desire to be busy, could scarcely give way to the wishes of the friends with whom I was associated.

INSOLENT (57/I)

Insolence is a lack of respect. It may be detected in patients during consultation, although few will admit to it. Look for an attitude of excessive casualness and confidence, the impertinence implicit in all the movements. This person is ill-mannered and completely lacking in modesty.

Materia Medica

CANTHARIS. An insolent and contradictory mood. Churlish mood.

INTROSPECTION (57/I)

Introspection is the scrutiny of one's own thoughts and feelings. People who have this symptom are absorbed in themselves, lost in thought. They seek out solitude in order to give themselves over to fantasy and dreams.

Boenninghausen combines 'Introversion' and 'Introspection' under the same heading in his *Repertory*. This happy association is the result of the indivisibility of both symptoms, since the introverted person is best characterised by his constant tendency to introspection. When a patient claims to be introverted, one must ask him to explain himself exactly. If he really means that he is taciturn, timid, reserved, misanthropic or that he represses aggressive feelings, then one should refer to the appropriate rubric in each case. If however the patient explains that he experiences a 'world within' and is at the same time reticent, uncommunicative, solitary and unsociable, this would indicate the presence of the symptom.

The psychological concept of introversion since Jung includes all the above qualities. In homoeopathy, though, one must identify every symptom the patient shows, even though each may overlap with others.

Practical Examples

'I shut myself off in my own little world, I like to be alone, I'm introverted, reticent, I find it hard to communicate.'

'I'm always lost in thought, very introverted, I'm not communicative. I don't like telling people things, I find it hard to strike up relationships.'

'My mind tends to wander, I become self-absorbed, lost in thought, introspective and reflective. I seem to spend more time in a dream world than in the real one. My husband says I'm introverted.'

Materia Medica

VIOLA TRICOLOR. Introspective, discontented with himself, distrustful of himself, especially of his future.

IRRESOLUTION (57/I) *unsure of how to act*

The indecision of the irresolute person thrives on doubt and hesitancy and is apparent in all aspects of his public and private life. The irresolute child does not know if he wants to play or to go for a walk, or do both at once. The indecisive student can never know what he wants to do in life; he weighs up the merits and drawbacks of one career against another, delays his decision, and once he has chosen, thinks that perhaps he was wrong. Then he does not know whether to change his job or carry on. The life of the irresolute person is a long series of deferred decisions and altered objectives. He can never decide whether his fiancée is the woman with whom he wants to spend his life, and even when he has made the decision, he will not go through with the marriage for a long time.

'Irresolution' may lie behind the symptom 'Postponing everything to next day' (*Synthetic Repertory* column 799).

Materia Medica

CALCAREA FLUORATA. Indecision.

CHAMOMILLA. Very anxious, everything that she undertakes is very unsatisfactory; she is irresolute, with flushes of heat in the palms.

COCA. Mood changeable, mostly very morose; irresolute, false and deceitful characters.

CUBEBA. Want of decision and will-power.

CUPRUM. Irresolute; satisfied with nothing; this only lasts as long as he is fretful.

FERRUM MAGNETICUM. Irresolute; he considers for a long time before commencing anything.

HYDROPHOBINUM. Undecided about little things.

IGNATIA. Inconstant, impatient, irresolute, quarrelsome, in recurring attacks every three or four hours.

IODUM. It is difficult to collect his senses, and he is irresolute.

KALI CARBONICUM. Irresolute mood.

LYCOPODIUM. Indecision and loss of confidence.

MAGNESIA MURIATICA. Irresolute.

NAJA. Sadness and irresolution.

NATRUM MURIATICUM. Irresolute at work; he could not see his way clearly.

NUX VOMICA. Irresolution; constant fickleness in his plans. Dawdles and is irresolute.

PETROLEUM. Very irresolute.

PHOSPHORUS. Discontented and irresolute.

PULSATILLA. Extreme irresolution. Shuns business, is irresolute, with sighing respiration and a feeling as if he were beside himself.

RUTA. Fretful, ill-humoured and irresolute.

SULPHUR. Indolent, irresolute.

TARAXACUM. Irresolution and dread of work, though it progresses well as soon as he undertakes it.

TARENTULA. Loss of memory, accompanied with good nature; changeable mind, tears, singing and irresoluteness.

IRRITABILITY, menses, before (59/II)

In order to be considered a true symptom this must occur every month, and the irritability must be severe.

When patients describe premenstrual tension they say they are 'nervy' or 'moody', 'impatient with the children', or 'more sensitive and touchy'. Some women have arguments or fights with their husbands and then realise that their next period is starting.

The symptom 'Sadness, menses, before' (77/I) is less frequently seen. It sometimes accompanies premenstrual tension.

Some women cry before every period but rarely do so at other times, for whatever reason. This is 'Weeping, menses, before' (94/I).

IRRITABILITY, waking, on (60/I)

Irritability on waking is a symptom found in men and women of all ages. Patients report that they 'get out of bed on the wrong side', and that they 'won't say anything for half an hour' and 'want to be left alone', and that their good humour returns only after a while.

One should check that the patient feels irritable not just on waking in the morning but also if he has a nap in the afternoon.

The symptom is present in children who are irritable when they are woken by someone else, but it would of course have more force if they were also irritable when they woke up by themselves.

JEALOUSY (60/I)

Great care must be taken in assessing this feeling, for it is very common, which detracts from its value as a symptom. Children and young couples frequently show signs of jealousy in one way or another, and in such cases it must exist to an unusual degree before one can consider it to be a true symptom.

One or more of the following characteristics should always be present:

- The jealousy is groundless. If a motive exists then it is not a symptom.
- The feeling is intense and obsessive.
- The jealousy causes feelings of suffering.
- The patient is reproachful, and this leads to rows with the partner.

Although there is always an element of envy in the jealous person, one should distinguish between the two feelings. A practical example will illustrate this point. A young woman whom I treated with Sepia told me at her first consultation that as a child she used to feel jealous of her brother. When I asked her why this was so, she replied, 'He was the boy and so they let him do things like come home late, or use bad language, whereas I was the 'baby' and had to play with my dolls.' In this case the main feeling was clearly one of envy, and not jealousy.

Materia Medica

ANANTHERUM. Ungovernable jealousy, everything causes jealousy.

LACHESIS. Towards evening a very unusual, almost crazy, jealousy, as foolish as it is irresistible.

NUX VOMICA. He quarrels, reproaches, scolds, insults from jealousy, mingled with unchaste expressions; soon afterwards howls and weeps aloud.

OPIUM. Appeared jealous and afraid of the people around.

JESTING (60/I); FACETIOUSNESS (41/II); HUMOROUS (52/I)

The joker is another well-known figure. He never misses a chance to tell a funny story. He leaves his own peculiar mark on everything. His aim is to amuse or to impress those around him.

When his jokes are witty and to the point the symptom is 'Witty' (95/I).

Jesting

Materia Medica

ARSENICUM. Inclines to jest in a malicious manner.

CAPSICUM. He is in a contented mood, is jocose, and sings, and still he becomes angry from the slightest causes. He makes jokes and utters witticisms.

CHLORALUM. Lively mood, with loud laughing and witty remarks.

COCCULUS. After a few hours, he became lively and jocose. (Curative action – Hahnemann.) Frolicsome, contented, joyous; he became witty and jocose.

CROCUS. Irresistible inclination to joke and laugh, with great prostration, and great dilatation of the pupils.

GLONOINUM. Unusually animated and talkative; great flow of thought and inclination to jest; for four hours.

IGNATIA. Merry and jesting mood. Incredible changes of mood; at one time he jokes and makes merry, at another he is lachrymose, alternating every three or four hours. / He jokes a few hours after he has been angry.

IPECACUANHA. Lively mood, he is inclined to talk, and even to joke.

LACHESIS. The more cause for fretfulness, the greater inclination for humour, jest, satire, and humorous fancies.

MENYANTHES. Keeps aloof from amusements (after twelve hours); half an hour afterwards is inclined to joke.

MERCURIALIS. Lively mood, inclined to sing and joke.

PETIVERIA. Disposed to laugh and jest.

SPONGIA. Pert, witty mood.

SUMBUL. Mirthfulness, smiling, good humour, wittily inclined; sympathy with suffering seems robbed of its pain. Mirthful, witty, inclined to gaiety; continued smiling; calm, contented; amorous.

TARENTULA. Desire to joke, to play, and to laugh; extreme gaiety. Lively and satisfied; disposition to joke.

LAMENTING, bemoaning, wailing (61/I)

The patient moans, cries and sighs as though in distress or great pain, but actually he does this only to arouse the sympathy of those around him.

Materia Medica

OPIUM. Lamentations and howling during the first hours.

LAUGHING, serious matters, over (62/I)

This is a curious symptom. Sometimes patients tell you that they laugh (usually involuntarily) in circumstances which are not funny and may even be distressing.

Practical Examples

'I crease up with laughter at serious events like funerals. On one occasion a baby caught his fingers in the door of a bus and I couldn't contain myself.'

'I don't cry easily. I get a tight feeling in my throat and then instead of crying I laugh. My behaviour can be peculiar – when I feel nervous I burst into laughter. Everybody tells me I'm strange.'

Materia Medica

ANACARDIUM. He laughs when he should be serious. When occupied with serious things he is obliged to laugh on account of a tickling at the pit of the stomach; when occupied with ludicrous things he is able to refrain from laughter.

LIE, never speaks the truth (62/II); LIAR (*Synthetic Repertory*, column 706)

Up to a certain point, lying is normal in small children. A 4-year-old child, for example, will invent or believe anything.

People may lie simply for the pleasure of lying, or in order to deceive other people or even themselves. There are those with a vivid imagination who mix fantasy with reality, who indulge their love of adventure with wonderful tales. Outrageous behaviour, histrionics and exaggeration are forms of lying specific to the hysterical character.

Patients rarely admit to being liars; usually it is the parents who will draw one's attention to this characteristic in their children. In such cases one must take into account the child's age, and whether the tendency to lie is constant and systematic.

A 24-year-old woman told me: 'Sometimes I say something and only realise what I said afterwards. I lie even though I don't want to. When people ask me where I'm from, I make up an answer. Sometimes I lie about my age. It's as though I were deceiving myself.'

LOQUACITY (63/I)

Loquacity is a symptom that is most commonly encountered in cases of hypermania. All conversation is swamped by a rapid and never-ending stream of words.

The talkative person is easy to identify. It is somewhat harder to elicit replies to the questions one puts to him, and he is well-nigh impossible to interrupt. From the homoeopath's point of view he is often an absolute pest, exhausting his patience as well as his other patients, should they be unfortunate enough to meet him in the waiting room.

Sometimes, in the context of a consultation, the talkativeness is a form of getting something off one's chest, a cathartic confession such as one might make to a priest. The symptom will be of more value if it is universal – that is, if the patient will talk to anyone at any time about anything at all.

LOVE, ailments, from disappointed (63/II)

Disappointed love may sometimes spark off a host of ailments for which the patient seeks treatment. It should not be confused with the symptom 'Grief, ailments, from' (51/I). The heading covers all kinds of emotional frustration.

The love may be for a partner, for a potential partner or for a member of the family. Great mental anguish and ailments due to the loss of the love of one or both parents is often typical of Natrum Muriaticum.

Some people avoid serious relationships for fear of subsequently losing a loved one. They are generally women who have suffered greatly as a result of a disappointment in love in the past, and who fear that it could happen again.

A 25-year-old woman came to me with epigastralgias, gastritis, migraines, nerves, depression and palpitations, going back some four years to when her parents had made her break off her engagement. She had not been able to put her fiancé out of her mind.

Related Symptom
'Chest, palpitation, heart, unrequited affections, from' (877/I)

Materia Medica

TARENTULA. Insanity on account of an unfortunate love. Great agitation. Great excitement.

TILIA. Lovesick; all his thoughts centred upon an ideal woman; in this reverie he was possessed by a sweet melancholy, which it was impossible to describe; every earthly sense seemed far away.

MAGNETIZED, desires to be (63/II)

In Hahnemann's time 'animal magnetism' (or 'Mesmerism' or 'hypnotism') was a widespread practice. Several paragraphs at the end of the *Organon* are devoted to a discussion of this subject.

The hypnotised person is typically very suggestible and there is a close link with the person who is hypnotising him. A modern-day equivalent of 'Magnetized, desires to be', might be seen in those children who need to be rubbed with a soft cloth on some part of the body before they will fall asleep. The symptom should not be confused with the desire to be massaged or rubbed, or improvement from this: 'Rubbing, amel.' (1368/I).

Practical Examples
'He likes to be caressed more than kissed or hugged. When we rub his head he behaves as though he's hypnotised.'
'He can't go to sleep until his head or back have been rubbed.'
'For many years he used to make himself go to sleep by rubbing some soft item of clothing of his mother's across his face.'

MALICIOUS (63/II)

It is important to note that Kent uses this as a general heading for several other closely-related symptoms: 'Resentment' (71/II), 'Revengeful' (75/I), 'Spiteful' (82/II) and 'Vindictive' (91/II).

As with other antisocial symptoms, the patient will not readily admit, even to himself, to being resentful. He may at most say, 'I don't bear grudges, but I've got a good memory', or 'I never forget'.

Other phrases one often comes across are: 'If someone offends me, then as far as I'm concerned he might as well not exist', or 'I don't feel any ill-will, I just feel sorry for him'. Again, the feeling must be intense and frequently experienced if it is to be a true symptom.

Such a patient's account of his relations with family and friends will reveal a lengthy history of malice towards one or more persons. Prompted by some slight, or an emotional frustration or a quarrel, in fact, by anything from a great hatred to a minor disagreement, the strength of the feeling does not diminish. Its distant origin is constantly brooded over. This person can neither forgive nor forget.

When treating children, bear in mind that their sense of time is different to that of adults. If one asks the parents how long their child's fits of anger last, a reply such as 'a few days' will indicate the presence of the symptom, for these few days are to a child what a few years are to an adult.

One Natrum Muriaticum patient illustrated how malice can originate in emotional frustration: 'I'm devoted to my wife, but if she was ever unfaithful to me, I would kill her. I could never forgive her.'

Resentment is often accompanied by a desire for revenge. 'Malicious' is the most appropriate rubric in such cases.

There is no great difference between 'Resentment' and 'Hatred' (51/I), though the former symptom is characterised by its persistence, and the latter by the suddenness with which it appears. In Kent's *Repertory*, 'Hatred' (51/I) is cross-referenced to 'Malicious'. In fact, all the remedies that appear under the rubric 'Hatred' (with the exception of Rhus Toxicodendron) are also included under 'Malicious'.

'Hatred' is typified by one patient who said, 'If my husband criticises me, I lash out at him. I hate him and wish he was dead.'

Materia Medica

COMOCLADIA. Combative, vindictive disposition for a whole week, and contempt for opponents.

HAEMATOXYLON. Spitefulness.

HYDRASTIS. Ill-humour; vindictiveness. Spiteful, angry disposition, with desire to snub anyone who differed in anything with me; lasting all day. Spitefulness and disposition to hit and knock things in general; disappeared towards evening.

MANGANUM. Embittered mood, implacable, and for a long time having a grudge against someone who had offended him.

NATRUM MURIATICUM. Hatred of people who had insulted him.

NITRICUM ACIDUM. Long-continued rancour, insensible to apologies and excuses.

OPIUM. Very vindictive at night.

PEDICULUS. Malicious, jeering temper.

SARRACENIA. Rancorous character, with great punctiliousness, especially when he feels sick.

SULPHUR. Numerous morbid and extremely disagreeable ideas cause rancour; but joyous thoughts (and melodies), mostly from the past, take possession of her; they throng one upon another so that she cannot free herself from them during the day, with neglect of business, worse in the evening in bed, when they prevent her from falling asleep.

TUSSILAGO FRAGRANS. Complaining mood, finding fault with everything, making spiteful remarks, the nature of which he does not himself recognise, and is astonished that others are offended at them; for this reason, when aware of their character, he remains silent for fear of offending his associates.

MEDDLESOME (64/I)

Poking one's nose into other people's affairs is a symptom that patients will hardly ever admit to. The sister of one patient told me, 'She loves to pry into other people's affairs. She listens behind doors and goes through people's handbags. She's very nosey.'

Another symptom that one learns of from relatives of the patient is 'Gossiping' (50/II). These people are as nosey as meddlesome patients, and their habit of talking about others indicates their tendency to lead vicarious lives.

MEMORY, weakness of (64/II)

The most common modalities are:

'Memory, weakness, expressing one's self, for' (64/II). This symptom is self-evident. At the consultation, the patient talks slowly and cannot find the words to construct his sentences. He does not know how to explain his symptoms.

'Memory, weakness, names, for proper' (65/I). This is the commonest modality. Some patients say they forget the names of members of the family, or friends, or even their own names (Medorrhinum).

'Memory, weakness, words, for' (65/I). This symptom applies when simple words in current usage are frequently forgotten.

MILDNESS (65/II); GENTLENESS (50/I)

There are two sides to this symptom. One is evident from the behaviour and bearing of the patient: meek and mild, polite and refined. The other refers to inherent docility and submissiveness. These are obedient and tolerant, rather characterless people. Both aspects may be found in the same patient.

Practical Examples
'I don't have much strength of character. I give in to people, let them do what they want.'
'I'm kind to a fault, I can't say no, I'm too docile and weak.'
'I always gave in to my husband. I was scared that he would leave me otherwise.'

Related Symptoms in the Synthetic Repertory
'Yielding disposition' (column 1102)
'Servile, obsequious, submissive' (column 909)

Materia Medica
CYCLAMEN. Gentle disposition, contented with himself.
IODUM. Mild, scrupulous, timid, with blunted sensibilities.
KALI CYANATUM. Gentle.
NATRUM MURIATICUM. Internal contentment, hope, gentleness (curative action).
SUMBUL. Mild, amiable, smiling.

MISANTHROPY (66/I)

The misanthrope is a hermit who seeks solitude in order to avoid humankind. He loathes and mistrusts everybody.

Materia Medica
CICUTA VIROSA. Want of confidence in mankind, with misanthropy; he forsook society, remained alone and reflected.
COPAIVA. Misanthropy.
CROTALUS HORRIDUS. Melancholy, misanthropic and indifferent, with sudden weakness, headache, heartache, and excessive diarrhoea.
CURARE. Aversion to society.
HYDROCOTYLE. Misanthropy.

KALI BICHROMICUM. Fear of people. / Apprehensiveness and aversion to society.

LEDUM. Discontented all day with his companions, which at last amounts to misanthropy.

LYCOPODIUM. Fear of people.

NATRUM CARBONICUM. Fear of people and fearfulness. He shuns mankind.

NATRUM MURIATICUM. Fear of people.

PHOSPHORUS. Was obliged to laugh against her will while she was sad.

RHUS GLABRA. Distaste for society; no desire to speak to anyone, or to be spoken to.

STANNUM. Aversion and dread of people.

TABACUM. Misanthropy.

MISCHIEVOUS (66/I)

This is a symptomatological gem that combines subtle aggression with ingenuity and vivaciousness. The mischievous person is a great prankster, who amuses himself or others by playing jokes on people or animals.

A mother described how her 'mischievous' 9-year-old daughter (Calcarea Carbonica) would tease the household pets, and how, on one occasion, she smeared mud all over the walls, and then said with a smile, 'I wonder who did that?'

Another patient told me that as a schoolboy he used to play tricks on the teachers with stink-bombs and plastic spiders, and stand buckets of water over the door to drench his classmates as they came into the room. Such people clearly derive a perverse sort of pleasure from these acts.

Materia Medica

AGARICUS. Fearless, menacing, mischievous frenzy; also, frenzy which causes the patient to assail and injure himself, with great exertion of power.

ALOE. The child is very much enlivened and vivacious, it plays and prattles uncommonly, with much mischievousness and laughter (from sucking Aloes).

BARYTA CARBONICA. Good humour becomes mischievousness.

CANNABIS INDICA. Full of fun and mischief, and laughs immoderately.

MOANING, groaning (67/I); WHINING (95/I)

The patient makes a piteous sound when he is suffering from pain, grief, distress, despair, etc.

This is often accompanied by the symptoms 'Lamenting, bemoaning, wailing' (61/I) and 'Complaining' (12/II), and usually occurs during sleep or attacks of fever, both of which are modalities in the *Repertory*.

Materia Medica

ARSENICUM. Loud wailing. Moaned grievously. She lies crouched in bed, groaning and moaning. She spends the night in moaning and groaning.

CHAMOMILLA. Moaning on account of a very trifling offence, which had happened a long time ago. Moaning and groaning on account of ill humour. Involuntary moaning, with heat of the face. / Piteous moaning of a child because he cannot have what he wants.

CHINA . Moaning, complaining, and screaming.

CICUTA VIROSA. Weeping, moaning, and howling.

HURA BRASILIENSIS. Every paroxysm of pain excites a nervous laugh, with moanings like those of a sick child.

HYDROCYANICUM ACIDUM. Occasionally moaning.

IPECACUANHA. Whining mood; must be carried about.

NUX VOMICA. She moans and groans piteously without any assignable cause.

OXALICUM ACIDUM. Moaning.

PHOSPHORUS. Patient apathetic; at times tossing about the bed and moaning (sixth day).

STRYCHNINUM. Loud groans, convulsive sobbing. Moaning. Loud moaning. Constant moaning, with complete consciousness.

SULPHURICUM ACIDUM. Constant moaning. Moaning very deeply.

VERATRUM ALBUM. He groans, is beside himself; does not know what to do with himself.

MOCKING (67/II); FACETIOUSNESS (41/II)

The mocker is a false humorist. There is always an element of aggression in him; mockery is a means of avoiding direct aggression. What he says is devious and deliberately ironic. The mocker aims to

96

humiliate and ridicule his adversary. His attitude is one of scorn which he hides in a smile.

Related Symptoms
'Irony, satire, desire for' (*Synthetic Repertory*, column 650)
'Jesting, malicious' (60/I)

MORAL feeling, want of (68/I)

This is an all-embracing symptom that applies to those who systematically commit immoral or anti-social acts. These people are indifferent to the rights and feelings of others (see 'Wicked disposition' (95/I) and 'Cruelty' 17/I)). They feel a need to cause harm; evil, for them, is an end in itself.

MORTIFICATION, ailments after (68/II); CHAGRIN (10/II)

This symptom will emerge spontaneously during the consultation, or else one can ask the patient what things move or affect him. Many illnesses such as duodenal ulcers and coronary thrombosis can have their origin in chagrin.

In 'Mortification', chagrin acts as an exciting cause or irritating factor which threatens the patient's health. The two classic examples are the employee who puts up with the continual bullying of his boss, and the wife who knows that her husband is unfaithful to her.

The mortified patient feels abused, humiliated and annoyed (see 'Indignation' (55/II).

Practical Examples
'For ten long years I put up with my husband; I knew he had been deceiving me right from the beginning. It ruined my health. He's a good-for-nothing, he never works.'
'At the time of the junta I was made redundant – I used to be the matron at a hospital. I felt so helpless, it hurt me terribly. I cried for a month and it gave me glaucoma.'
'I take things to heart. I turn my grievances over in my mind and then I feel terrible.'

Materia Medica

FORMICA. Sudden and unexpected return of sense of mortification and grief, with vivid recollection of circumstances long since passed, which had caused great mortification and pain, and which had rendered several years of his life unhappy; this was caused by the transactions of a near relative; this grief continues, and manifests itself whenever he is not occupied.

Kent's Materia Medica

COLOCYNTHIS. Colocynth produces a state in the nervous system like that found in individuals who have for years been labouring under annoyances and vexations. A man whose business affairs have been going wrong becomes irritable, and nervous exhaustion follows. A woman who must watch her unfaithful husband night and day to keep him away from other women gradually assumes a sensitive, irritable state of mind, and is upset by the least provocation. This is the state of the Colocynth prover.

OBSTINATE (69/I); HEADSTRONG (51/II); STUBBORN (84/I)

Obstinacy is a well-known characteristic. It should be differentiated from 'Contradiction, is intolerant of' (16/II), 'Defiant' (17/II) and 'Positiveness' (69/II).

The symptom has many synonyms: stubborn, headstrong, stiff-necked, pig-headed, dogged, pertinacious. An obstinate person is someone who sticks to an opinion or idea to the bitter end. Nothing can convince him of his error or induce him to change his point of view. He just will not budge an inch.

Another manifestation of this symptom is perseverance. This applies to an obstinate person with a strong will who works tirelessly and tenaciously to achieve his aims. He keeps his objectives clearly in view, and any obstacles he meets only serve to redouble his efforts and concentration.

Materia Medica

ARNICA. Obstinate and headstrong resistance to other people's opinions.
CALCAREA CARBONICA. Obstinate disposition. / Obstinate, depressed mood.

CAMPHORA. Desire to dispute; self-willed.

CAPSICUM. Obstinate, and cries out.

CARBO ANIMALIS. Obstinate; no one could do anything to suit him.

CAUSTICUM. Furiously opinionated and quarrelsome.

CHAMOMILLA. Fretful, out of humour, and obstinate, even to quarrelling, at the start of the menstrual flow.

CHELIDONIUM. Obstinacy.

DROSERA. Obstinate in the execution of his carefully-laid plans.

HEPAR SULPHURIS. Extremely fretful and obstinate.

IGNATIA. He is discontented, morose, and obstinate towards evening; no one can do anything right or please him.

IPECACUANHA. Extremely inclined to be obstinate and fretful.

KALI IODATUM. Stubborn obstinacy.

LYCOPODIUM. He can hardly conceal an internal obstinacy.

MURIATICUM ACIDUM. Obstinate, fretful; unwilling to take up any work; in the evening.

NITRICUM ACIDUM. Peevish, with a sad and obstinate mood, with restlessness, so that she does not know where to turn.

PHOSPHORIC ACIDUM. Obstinate about everything.

PHOSPHORUS. Obstinate .

SILICEA. Nervous excitement. / The child becomes obstinate and headstrong. / Obstinate.

SULPHUR. Obstinate and lachrymose at the time of the morning stool. Can think of nothing to be thankful for; is obstinate and unyielding without knowing why. / So obstinate and morose that he answers no one, and will tolerate no one about him; cannot obtain quickly enough whatever he desires.

OCCUPATION, amel. (69/I)

Improvement from busying oneself is a common symptom. The improvement may be physical or mental. It is mostly expressed as an inability to be inactive; these people cannot bear to be idle even for a minute. In a frenzy they hurl themselves into one task after another without a break. This compulsive need to be occupied often leads them to do things without really being involved in the task. They will read anything that comes to hand, no matter whether it is interesting or not; the point is to read more, not to 'waste' a single moment. Manual activities are better still – knitting is the mainstay of many hyperactive women. Many such patients knit in the waiting room, on the bus, or while watching television.

The symptom should not be confused with 'Busy' (10/I) and 'Industrious' (56/I).

Practical Examples

'I can't bear to be idle. I've always got things to do and if not then I'll go and find something to keep me busy.'

'I'm not happy unless I'm knitting, even if I'm watching television.'

'When I get depressed I busy myself so as not to dwell on things.'

'I'm nervous and restless, I don't stop for a second, I have to keep busy otherwise I would start to despair.'

'I'm very active, I'm always doing something around the house, painting or mending. If I don't have anything to do then I'll find something, or else I wouldn't feel right. I hate to waste time.'

'I have always been very active, I'm always knitting or sewing something, I can't bear to be idle and to waste my time. If I don't have anything to do I feel very lazy and get depressed.'

'I always need to be occupied. If I'm watching television I'll be knitting or sewing at the same time – I feel as though if I didn't do that I'd be wasting my time.'

'I'm hyperactive, even when I'm on holiday I find things to do. If not I get worried and depressed.'

OFFENDED, easily (69/I)

People who have this symptom are susceptible to taking offence at trifling things or harmless jokes, to which they may react with irritability or even violence. They may be insecure people, or have an overblown sense of honour, which can lead to a feeling of malice when slighted.

The symptom 'Irritability, takes everything in bad part' (60/I) should be combined with 'Offended, easily', for the purposes of repertorisation.

POSITIVENESS (69/II)

This is a variant form of obstinacy with distinctive characteristics. The symptom is essentially one of excessive self-confidence, of certainty in word and deed. We are not concerned here with a normal characteristic – symptoms, to be of significance, must be outstanding to a pathological degree. In 'Positiveness', the capacity to doubt does not exist. Nothing is worth discussing; he is always right and has a monopoly on the truth.

Those who claim to be very sure of themselves often have an underlying feeling of insecurity. However, this mechanism does not exist in 'Positiveness'. Such a person never suffers from timidity, anticipatory nerves or cowardice, etc.

A symptom closely linked both to obstinacy and to positiveness is 'Pertinacity'(69/II), when the patient stubbornly sticks to opinions or decisions.

In Boenninghausen's *Repertory* the headings 'Dogmatic' and 'Positiveness' contain the same remedies: Camphora, Causticum, Ferrum Metallicum, Lachesis and Mercurius Vivus.

Practical Example
'I'm headstrong, I find it hard to listen to other people's opinions. People say I'm too sure of myself, that I never doubt the truth of anything I say.' (33-year-old woman)

POSTPONING everything to next day (*Synthetic Repertory*, column 799)

This symptom may be associated with 'Indolence', or it may stem from a fear of undertaking things, or of failure. The fewer the reasons for this kind of behaviour, the greater its value as a symptom.

Practical Examples
'I tend to put things off; I've been meaning to go and learn to play tennis for two years now. I leave things like buying clothes and taking the car to be serviced much longer than I ought to.'
'I never do things I don't want to do. I put them off until I can't avoid them any more.'
'He postpones things until the last possible minute, even though he knows that it gets him into trouble.'

PRECOCITY (69/II)

A precocious child is one who develops mental or physical qualities in advance of the age at which they normally appear: one who can read well at three years, or stand up, with support, at the age of four months, or who begins teething even earlier than this. Care should be taken in evaluating this symptom as parents are understandably apt to exaggerate their children's abilities.

Calcarea Carbonica appears in the *Synthetic Repertory* under this heading (column 800) and is taken from Kent's *Lectures on Homoeopathic Materia Medica*. It should be noted that according to Kent, Calcarea Carbonica is only for religious precocity.

Paschero has added Carcinosin to this symptom; in my experience, this is the remedy that is most often indicated.

QUARRELSOME (70/I); CONTENTIOUS (16/II); SCOLDING (78/I)

A quarrelsome person is someone who starts rows and looks for trouble. He may merely be abusive (see 'Abusive' (1/II)) or actually become violent (see 'Fight, wants to' (48/I)).

In Kent's *Repertory* 'Scolding' is cross-referenced to 'Quarrelsome'. Scolding, or telling people off for no good reason, is difficult to distinguish from 'Complaining' (12/II), and includes a measure of 'Intolerance' (*Synthetic Repertory*, column 648).

Although the symptom 'Fight, wants to' applies to cases of physical rather than verbal aggression, it should be combined with 'Quarrelsome' for the purposes of repertorisation.

RESERVED (72/I)

The reserved person does not show his feelings or betray his thoughts.

He may confide only in one intimate friend; but equally he may not even confide in his beloved wife. One cannot know his thoughts; sometimes he does not even know them himself.

Such people never talk about themselves and are very hard to get to know. In some cases they may hide behind a shield of talkativeness, but in general they are taciturn.

Practical Examples

'Emotionally I'm fairly stable. I tend to keep things to myself. I give the impression of being secure but inside I'm actually rather frightened, although nobody knows this because I'm very reserved.'
(A mother said of her 10-year-old girl): 'When she starts talking no one can stop her, but she never shows her true feelings.'
'I'm introverted, I don't tell secrets.'
'I'm reserved, an introvert. I don't express my emotions or anger, or talk about things that are important to me.'
(A mother, of her 12-year-old): 'She is very timid, very introverted, she finds it hard to show her feelings or to open up, she doesn't confide in us.'
'I'm not very chatty and wouldn't tell anyone anything intimate.'
'I keep my own counsel. I don't like to lay myself open.'

Materia Medica

PLATINUM. Reserved, cold, absent-minded in the company of friends, in the open air.

RUDENESS (75/I)

This symptom is related to 'Insolent', and the characteristics of both are similar. The rude person is impolite and coarse in word and deed. Like the insolent person he has absolutely no consideration for anyone else, but the rude person adds a dash of crudeness and bad taste. The symptom is to be seen most clearly in ignorant and uncouth people.

The symptom 'Rudeness, ailments from' (75/I) is of great value. Those with a particular susceptibility to rudeness are more deeply hurt by the way in which people address them than by what they actually say.

Practical Examples

'I get upset if people don't speak to me nicely. I'm very easily hurt.'
'I'm a rather sensitive plant and feel awful if someone raises their voice at me. I like to be treated with consideration.'
'I'm very susceptible to how people behave towards me. I take offence easily and don't like it when people speak to me in a nasty tone of voice.'
'I really can't stand being shouted at, or having people be rude to me. I like considerate people.'

'It's not so much what they say as how they say it. That's what matters. I feel deeply hurt when people use bad language.'

SADNESS, cloudy weather (76/II)

There is just one remedy for this symptom, and that is Ammonium Carbonicum. It is best to combine it with the more general rubric 'Cloudy weather agg.' (1348/II), which covers a large group of remedies. Sadness during cloudy weather is a symptom that one frequently encounters. In order to be valid the patient must experience it whenever the sky is overcast. Naturally it should be discarded if a logical explanation exists. One patient said that he became depressed on cloudy days because he associated them with rain, which reminded him of the house where he was born. Its roof used to leak, and this put him in mind of the poverty of his early days.

SCORN, ailments from (78/I)

This refers to people who are particularly susceptible to being slighted or treated in a scornful manner.

Practical Examples
'I can't help taking offence very easily, and it takes me a long while to get over it.'
'If someone snubs or slights me I fall ill.'
'I'm very easily hurt if someone treats me with contempt. I feel as though any remark made about me is always a nasty one.'

Materia Medica
CHAMOMILLA. Disposed to anger, scorn and quarrelsomeness. / Morose, inclined to scorn.
CICUTA VIROSA. Contempt and scorn for mankind; he avoided them, abhorred their follies excessively, and his disposition seemed to tend towards misanthropy; he withdrew himself into solitude.
COMOCLADIA. Self-complacent thoughts and contempt of others.
GUAIACUM. Contemptuousness.
IPECACUANHA. Ill-humoured, quiet, retired in himself, scorning every-thing. Morose mood that scorns everything, and desires also that others shall not appreciate or value anything.

NATRUM MURIATICUM. Scornful, ill-natured, excited.

NUX VOMICA. Scornful, peevish, inclined to be angry.

PLATINUM. Contemptuous, pitiful. Looking down upon people usually venerated, with a kind of casting them off, in paroxysms, against her will.

SPONGIA. Scornful, obstinate, ill-humoured.

SECRETIVE (78/I)

Secretive people keep quiet about things or hide their thoughts, feelings and intentions. The symptom is difficult to distinguish from 'Reserved' (72/I), but whereas the secretive person is always obsessed with hiding something, this is not necessarily true of the reserved patient.

SELFISHNESS (78/I)

The egoist thinks only of himself. All that matters are his own needs and his own well-being; he overlooks the interests of other people. He finds it impossible to share. He gives nothing of himself, not even his time, which is dedicated to his own concerns. The selfish child will eat his sweets alone and hide the rest from his friends so that he will not have to share them. Although his toys belong to him alone, he also wants to have the ones that belong to his brother and sister. Sharing is a concept he does not understand.

The unscrupulous person who takes advantage of other people for his own ends is also selfish.

Related Symptoms
'Indifference, others, toward' (55/I)
'Indifference, welfare of others, to' (55/II)

Practical Examples
'I'm selfish, I take what I need without a thought for other people; everything revolves around myself.'
'I had an argument with my wife because she lent the hair drier to a friend. I needed it and it wasn't there. It's mine, not hers.'
'My wife, who is a psychologist, was telling me about a patient of hers, but I quickly lost interest and wanted to get on with something else. She accused me of not listening to her, of always being self-obsessed.'

'Marcello (his mother told me) always does what he wants to, he hogs the television and no one else can watch another channel. He never thinks of others before himself.'

'I'm very possessive, I don't lend my tools to anyone, and I wouldn't even lend my car to my wife.'

SENSITIVE, noise, slightest (79/I)

The dripping of a tap, the noise of the wind, the ticking of a watch, the buzz of a fly; all these little noises get on the nerves of patients with this symptom. They hear them all and find them intensely irritating.

SENSITIVE, sensual impressions, to (79/I)

This symptom must be present to an exaggerated degree before it can be taken into consideration. It applies to those people who are constantly thinking about the pleasures of the senses and how to satisfy them. They like to eat and drink well, enjoy good music and take much pleasure in sex. They love to tingle with every possible pleasant sensation.

They make a cult of these inclinations and devote much time, imagination and energy to them.

A female patient said, 'I am very sensual, I'm very fond of music, of colours, shapes, dancing, drawing, physical pleasures. I enjoy tastes and eat slowly in order to savour them.'

The rubric 'Gourmand' (*Synthetic Repertory*, column 565) is a related symptom which refers to people who enjoy sumptuous meals and who delight in lots of good food.

SENTIMENTAL (79/II)

A sentimental person is someone with an exaggerated sensibility that arouses different feelings in him – of rapture, joy, delight, grief, sadness, and so on. In evaluating the importance of this symptom one must take into account the force of the stimulus involved.

The stimulus is likely to be a pleasant one such as a sunset, a sunrise, a landscape, a plant, or some other natural thing. Another way of expressing the symptom is by conferring a private symbolic value on material objects that evoke feelings of past happiness. Such people keep old bus tickets, cinema programmes and other souvenirs of happy times shared with a loved one (Pulsatilla). Sentimental by nature, they are easily moved to tears or touched by anything, however trivial, because their minds are already full of emotional scenes.

The symptom may cover others, such as 'Sympathetic' (86/I), 'Homesickness' (51/I), or 'Affectionate' (4/II), which do not by themselves always imply sentimentality.

Materia Medica

ALCOHOL. A sanguine and choleric temperament grows sentimental and passionate; they show the greatest inclination to love and voluptuousness.

ANTIMONIUM CRUDUM. Continual condition of ideal love and ecstatic longing for some ideal female being, which wholly filled his fancy; more when walking in the open pure air than in the room; this symptom disappeared after a few days, the sexual desire apparently diminished at the same time.

COFFEA CRUDA. Lively fancies; full of plans for the future; contrary to his custom is very much charmed by the beauties of nature, descriptions of which are related to him.

LACHESIS. Great irritability; soothing poetry moved him to immoderate weeping; he was obliged to cry for joy; as for example, when reading in Schiller's *Wilhelm Tell*, he could not proceed; an unmanly rapture compelled him to desist; in exciting scenes he broke into tears, and so on for a great many days; after much crying, pain above the eyes.

PSORINUM. Very sentimental.

SERIOUS (79/II); EARNESTNESS (39/I); GRAVITY (50/II); SOLEMN (81/II)

The people in this group are always and on every occasion circumspect, serious and formal. They are never cheerful, and never laugh at or make jokes. The opposite symptom is 'Frivolous' (50/I).

Materia Medica

ARSENICUM. Great seriousness.

CHINA. Earnest mood.

CINA. Great earnestness and sensitiveness; he is offended at the slightest joke.

CYCLAMEN. Although previously lively, he now became suddenly very earnest and somewhat fretful; after some time he became again lively, soon again ill-humoured.

FERRUM. I am inclined to attribute great importance to trifles, and am generally in an unusually earnest mood, without external cause.

GRATIOLA. Earnest, reflective mood.

HYDROPHOBINUM. Felt unusually serious.

IGNATIA. Quiet, earnest, melancholy; cannot be induced to talk or be cheerful; with flat, watery taste to all food, and little appetite.

LEDUM. Great earnestness all day; everything which happened to him was viewed thoughtfully and seriously.

ORIGANUM. Her disposition was very much affected; after the fifth or sixth day she became earnest, fearful, silent, sad, discontented, despairing, and weary of life.

PHOSPHORICUM ACIDUM. Sad, earnest, discouraged only when walking in the open air, the farther he walks the more it increases; in the house it gradually disappears, and he becomes more lively.

PLATINUM. Very earnest and taciturn the first day, on the next day she made jokes and laughed at everything.

SENECIO. Evening, in a very meditative mood, very serious, disposition to think of the past and future.

STAPHYSAGRIA. Earnest mood, quietly busy with himself, speaks very little.

SULPHURIC ACIDUM. Sedate, earnest condition of mind.

THUJA. Remarkably earnest mood in a young girl. / Very earnest frame of mind in spite of the cheerfulness of those around him, in the evening.

TILIA. Earnest, reflective mood.

VALERIANA. Seriousness.

SIGHING (80/II)

This is a minor but nevertheless interesting symptom which may be observed directly; at intervals the patient will sigh deeply. When questioned he will say he always does it, and that sometimes his friends tease him about it. It may or may not relate to depressive conditions.

SLOWNESS (81/I)

This patient is slow in everything he does. He is generally passive and quiet. The homoeopath will recognise the symptom by the patient's leisurely speech, or by the time he takes to put his clothes back on after a medical examination. Sometimes mothers tell you that their children take an eternity to get ready for school in the morning.

SYMPATHETIC (86/I)

A sympathetic person is able to enter into or share the problems of another person, to feel them as though they were his own. He is moved merely by reading or hearing about suffering. It should be noted that there is no firm agreement on the definition of this symptom – some authorities maintain that it cannot exist unless the patient is actively engaged in trying to find a solution to the problem, while others claim that the feeling by itself is sufficient.

Sympathy is prompted by the slightest things – a stray dog, the sight of a bird that has fallen out of its nest, and so on – and the suffering the patient feels at such sights persists after the event. The degree of pain felt must be high before this natural attribute can be considered a homoeopathic symptom. In certain cases one can rule it out immediately; for example, if someone who has himself known poverty feels pity for someone in similar circumstances, that in fact is a form of self-pity. There is always an aspect of altruism in true sympathy, and it extends beyond family and friends to include strangers. The symptom generally emerges in response to the question, 'What sort of things move you?'

Do not confuse sympathy with impressionability. If a person is upset by an accident, or the death or illness of another person, this symptom is usually 'Horrible things, sad stories affect her profoundly' (52/I).

Materia Medica
ALCOHOL. A sulky man becomes social and sympathetic.
CARLSBAD. His nerves are so much affected that the sorrows of others cause him to weep easily.
CAUSTICUM. Excessively sympathetic; she is beside herself with weeping and sobbing, and cannot be contented when listening to accounts of the hardships of others.
MANCINELLA. Feelings of tenderness and deep compassion.

NUPHAR LUTEUM. Excessive moral sensibility, giving one great pain on witnessing the sufferings of animals.

PHOSPHORUS. Ill-humour during the last days of the proving; she became exceedingly sensitive to the crying of a child, which affected her very unpleasantly, which had never before been the case.

THEORIZING (87/I), AIR castles (1/II)

The theorist is easy to identify when he comes for consultation. He leaves his stamp on everything he says. His account is a long list of examples and explanations.

He is remarkable for his inclination to learning and knowledge, of which he makes a cult. He lives on a plane of thought aloof from the real world. His mind, emotions and will are absorbed by the abstract.

Theorists prefer to think rather than to act. They are 'armchair experts' on many different subjects, and are usually incapable of solving practical problems. People who 'build castles in the air', who make plans that they have no hope of fulfilling, are also 'theorists'.

Practical Examples
(A woman said of her husband): 'I tell him that he has delusions of grandeur because he's always making pie-in-the-sky plans, like buying a house by the sea.' The husband's reply was: 'It costs nothing to dream.'
'I make totally unrealistic, crazy plans.'

The symptom 'Plans, making many' (69/II) may also be present in some cases, as the following examples show:
'I'm always making lots of plans. I ought to talk less and do more because they never leave the drawing board.'
'I'm a dreamer, I've always got my head in the clouds, I'm very idealistic.'

Materia Medica
CHINA. He has many ideas, a variety of things occupy his mind; he builds castles in the air. He makes many plans and reflects upon their execution; many ideas crowd upon him at once. His head is full of many plans which he would like to execute, in the evening.
COFFEA CRUDA. Lively fancies; full of plans for the future; contrary to his custom is very much charmed by the beauties of nature, descriptions of which are related to him.

NATRUM CARBONICUM. His mind is mostly busy with apprehensions of the future; he often makes plans for half an hour at a time, as if it would go wrong with him.

SEPIA. Dullness of comprehension; inability to collect or express his thoughts; constantly building castles in the air or running on future events.

SULPHUR. Greatly inclined to philosophical and religious reveries.

TIMIDITY (88/II); SHY (80/I); EMBARRASSED (39/II)

Timidity is a characteristic which may be evident from the patient's posture and attitude during the consultation. But sometimes the homoeopath may be surprised to hear the patient describe himself as timid, and say that he would not even have the courage to ask a passer-by what the time was, nor dare go into a shop to find out the price of something.

A 30-year-old Silica woman, married and with children, came to me essentially because she felt that her marked timidity was holding her back in life. Although her family background had been stable and she had made a successful career, she claimed to feel 'paralysed' and struck dumb at meetings, even relatively unimportant ones, and experience great discomfort as a result. She avoided getting into lifts with people she knew. She recalled that as a child she would hide behind her mother whenever anyone tried to talk to her.

One should establish whether a reticent and sober person is also timid (see 'Reserved' (72/I)).

An interesting modality is 'Timidity, appearing in public' (89/I). Some people feel shy only when in groups, particularly large ones; they avoid attending meetings, sit in the last row in lecture halls and wish that the earth would swallow them up should they have to speak out themselves.

Another important sub-rubric is 'Timidity, bashful' (89/I). This refers to the person who blushes when he has made a mistake or feels humiliated.

Materia Medica

AURUM. Timidity.

CARBO ANIMALIS. Shy and fearful mood.

COFFEA TOSTA. Timidity, and fear of sudden death; this fear sometimes causes trembling from head to foot.

FERRUM PHOSPHORICUM. At one time this afternoon cross words by another person about an absent stranger created a feeling of momentary shrinking and timidity.

IGNATIA. Fearfulness, timidity; she has no confidence in herself, gives up everything.

IODUM. Disposition mild, scrupulous and timid, with blunted sensibilities.

KALI BROMATUM. His character also had undergone a radical change, from having been very frank and brave, he had become excessively timid, and suspicious of every trifling circumstance.

MOSCHUS. It made her feel quiet and self-possessed; no fear of anything, is usually nervous and timid.

NATRUM CARBONICUM. Great timidity. He is very timid, and starts at the slightest noise.

PHOSPHORUS. Mental depression, and a most uncommon fearfulness or timidity, with a great sense of fatigue.

PIPER METHYSTICUM. Want of vigour, timid, apprehensive, during day.

PLATINUM. Great anxiety, with violent palpitation when attempting to talk in company, so that talking was difficult.

SULPHUR. Unusually timid.

TABACUM. From having been one of the most healthy and fearless of men, he had become sick all over and as timid as a girl; he could not even present a petition in Congress, much less say a word concerning it; though he had long been a practising lawyer, and had served much in a legislative body.

TOUCH things, impelled to (89/II)

People with this symptom seem to think that everything around them must continually be inspected by hand.

Children, at the consultation, touch everything: pictures, books, the prescription pad, the lamp, the scales, the sphygmomanometer – the lot. They sorely try the patience of the homoeopath, who is not spared the restless touch of the children's fingers.

UNFORTUNATE, feels (91/II)

This is a rather difficult symptom to define, and none of the materia medicas shed much light on it. It is most often found in women. One patient told me, 'I feel quite wretched', and when I asked her to explain what she meant she replied that it was not something that she could put into words. Occasionally people will venture that they have a feeling that they are 'useless', 'worthless' or 'a nonentity'. (See 'Delusions, wretched, thinks she looks, when looking in a mirror' (35/II).)

There is a profound feeling of misfortune, of being unlucky and unhappy, of being contemptible in both body and mind.

The symptom 'Delusions, unfortunate, that he is' (34/I), is closely related to 'Unfortunate, feels', and has the same remedies.

Related Symptoms
'Confidence, want of self' (13/II)
'Delusions, wretched, thinks she looks, when looking in a mirror' (35/II). There is little difference between feeling wretched and feeling unfortunate. When the symptom is unclear, both should be used for the purposes of repertorisation.
'Pities herself' (69/II)
'Weeping, pitied, if he believes he is' (94/I)

Practical Examples in which one or more of these symptoms appear
'I feel wretched, I think I'm worthless, everything I do and say is useless.'
'I feel very sorry for myself, I'm nothing.'
'I feel like a piece of shit, nothing at all. I feel quite empty and worthless inside. I just can't make a success of myself. It's made me very bitter, I'm tired of being so pitiful.'
'Sometimes I feel wretched and then I feel sorry for myself.'
'I'm full of self-pity, I feel very sorry for myself. If I cry in front of my husband I feel awful, really miserable.'

Materia Medica
AGARICUS. She is vexed with herself and pities herself.
CAUSTICUM. Anxiety the whole day, as if he had done something bad, or apprehended it, or as if he had been unfortunate.
CUBEBA. Regards himself as more of an invalid than he really is; fancies he is very unfortunate.
IPECACUANHA. Ill-humoured; he thinks that he is very unhappy.
MERCURIUS SOLUBILIS. Much wretchedness and dejection of spirits, with diarrhoea.
NATRUM MURIATICUM. She often looks into the mirror, and imagines that she looks wretched.

SARSAPARILLA. The soul is affected inordinately by the pains; the mind is depressed, the mood dull; he feels wretched, and moans involuntarily.

SEPIA. Gloominess; she feels unfortunate, without cause. / The greatest loathing of life; it seemed to him as if he could not endure so miserable an existence any longer, and as if he would pine away if he did not kill himself. / Memory so poor I cannot remember the least thing, and it makes me feel very miserable.

STAPHYSAGRIA. She was full of grief all day; she grieved over her condition and wept; nothing in the world pleased her.

UNOBSERVING (91/II)

This symptom signifies an inability to notice things, rather than, as some have thought, an attitude of defiance. Such patients are inattentive and easily distracted. Paschero combined the rubric with 'Forgetful', 'Absent-minded', and 'Heedless'.

Materia Medica
CAUSTICUM. Inattentive and distracted.
NATRUM CARBONICUM. Completely inattentive.
PETROLEUM. Hypochondriacal while walking in the open air, inattentive in conversation, etc.
SEPIA. No desire to work, inattentive, absent-minded.

VIOLENT (91/II)

This is a common symptom which scarcely needs to be defined. Note also 'Anger, violent' (3/I). The modality 'Violent deeds, rage, leading to' (91/II) is particularly useful. This is the most blatant form of aggression. The classic example of the symptom is the person who does not hesitate to use his fists on the slightest provocation.

The most violent types of aggression fall into the category of mania, and should be sought under the symptom headings 'Rage, fury' (70/II) and 'Wildness' (95/I).

Specific forms of aggression may be directed either at others or at oneself.

Symptoms Involving Violence Towards Others
'Biting' (9/II)
'Cut others, desires to' (17/I)
'Kicks' (60/II)
'Spits in faces of people' (82/II)
'Striking' (84/I)
'Throws things at persons' (88/II)

Symptoms Involving Self-inflicted Violence
'Injure, fears to be left alone, lest he should himself' (56/I)
'Killed, desires to be' (61/I)
'Pull one's hair, desires to' (70/I)
'Striking, knocking his head against wall' (84/I)
'Suicidal disposition' (85/I)

WEEPING (92/II)

This is one of the most important groups among the mental symptoms. The chief modalities are:

WEEPING, admonitions, cause (93/I)

This should be combined with 'Weeping, remonstrated with, when' (94/II) for the purposes of repertorisation. Weeping when admonished occurs principally in children, in whom a telling-off may be feared more than a smack. A child who cries when scolded may be expressing fear of being rejected. A 6-year-old girl said 'You don't love me any more' every time she was told off. One mother said of her daughter, 'She cries and then gets frightened that she'll get a telling-off, so she tries very hard to make up.'

WEEPING, causeless (93/I)

This modality occurs in depressive patients, although I once came across it in a patient who was not sad. He told me, 'When I started to get problems with my digestion I would burst into tears for no reason at all. Nobody could understand it; I certainly couldn't. People thought my marriage must be breaking up.'

Materia Medica

GRAPHITES. He was obliged to weep, without cause, in the evening.

HURA BRASILIENSIS. Causeless weeping, followed by nervous laughter.

KALI CARBONICUM. Great sadness; is obliged to weep without cause, in the evening.

NATRUM MURIATICUM. Sad and weeping mood, without cause.

RHUS TOXICODENDRON. Sad, begins to weep without knowing why.

STAPHYSAGRIA. She will hear or know nothing from anyone; she wraps up her face and weeps aloud without cause.

SULPHUR. Greatly inclined to weep without cause. At 11 a.m. impatience, anger, vexation, inclination to weep, without cause; this state of feeling lasts all the rest of the day, towards noon, the same feelings of weariness and impatience as the day before.

WEEPING, easily (*Synthetic Repertory*, column 1078)

This symptom does not appear in Kent's *Repertory*. It applies to the archetypal cry-baby, who cries in any circumstance.

WEEPING, involuntary (93/II)

Patients sometimes say that they cry when they don't want to. The crying fits are sudden and uncontrollable. The opposite symptom is 'Sadness, weep, cannot' (78/II).

Materia Medica

ALUMINA. The boy weeps constantly against his will, for half an hour.

IGNATIA. Involuntary weeping for three days.

KREOSOTUM. Music, or anything else that caused emotional excitement, she took very much to heart, and could not refrain from weeping.

MERCURIUS SOLUBILIS. Almost involuntary weeping, followed by relief.

NATRUM MURIATICUM. She was involuntarily obliged to weep.

PLATINUM. Very lachrymose and fretful; she often wept involuntarily, which relieved her.

SARRACENIA. Laughing and involuntary crying.

WEEPING, telling of her sickness, when (94/II)

This symptom may obviously be observed directly during the consultation. The weeping must seem an inappropriate response to the emotional content of the patient's words, and should occur during subsequent consultations. One patient said, 'I have a compulsion to tell everyone what's wrong with me, and then I start to cry.'

WEEPING, thanked, when (94/II)

This modality is covered by only one remedy, Lycopodium, which is however a grade three. This becomes a very important keynote when the remedy covers the totality of the patient's symptomatology. Crying when thanked implies a special sensibility to gratitude which involves feelings of respect and self-esteem.

Practical Examples

On being asked what sort of things stirred his emotions, a Lycopodium patient replied, 'I'm always very moved when people thank me, or when they're grateful to me. I feel delighted, and so overwhelmed that I have to keep a grip on myself in order not to cry.'

'Going into teaching was such a wonderful thing, it's so noble, I get more out of it than my pupils do. I am always moved to tears when at the end of the year my work is publicly acknowledged.'

Materia Medica

LYCOPODIUM. Extremely sensitive mood; she cries about being thanked.

WEEPING, trifles, at (94/II)

As one may suppose, this is a symptom mainly found in children. For the purposes of repertorisation it should generally be combined with 'Weeping, at the least worry, children' (94/II).

Practical Examples

'She cries over nothing at all. She even cries when she asks for something.' (5-year-old girl)

'She's a cry-baby. She cries if I tell her to hurry up, or if she can't get her hair to look right, or if she can't play a game properly.' (7-year-old girl)

'There's nothing that doesn't seem to make her cry. If she can't do up her laces or find her pencil her first reaction is to cry.' (6-year-old girl)

'I cry about the silliest things. If my mother tells me my bedroom is in a mess it makes me cry.' (16-year-old girl)

WICKED disposition (95/I)

This is an extreme form of maliciousness, found in perverse and abnormal people who damage the social fabric and do great harm to the lives of other people. The symptom is prevalent among criminals, murderers, thieves and swindlers. Evil people show no sign of guilt or regret.

Materia Medica

CUBEBA. Furious insanity, with wickedness; he breaks everything within his reach, out of sheer malice.

CURARE. Irascibility, wicked disposition; desires to lie in wait in order to assault others, and even to kill and rob them.

SARRACENIA. Madness, with wickedness and fury, or good humour and extreme complacency.

Case Studies

Author's Note: The following six case studies are the unedited transcripts of initial consultations held before colleagues during clinical classes. They are intended to demonstrate how the homoeopath may start the case, and how symptoms can come to light during the patient's first account of his or her complaint. They are not presented as case histories as such. I saw three of the patients a second time, and comment briefly on what they told me then. The other three were each subsequently treated by another homoeopath and I did not see them again.

The reader will notice that not all the symptoms presented by the patient during the consultation are actually considered at the repertorisation stage. Why are some more important than others – is it a matter of intuition and experience, or is there a more systematic reason why this should be so? My view is that the repertorisation should be based on the 'minimum syndrome of maximum value', encapsulating the dilemma or disease-state of the patient. Besides this, symptoms must fulfil a set of conditions if they are to rank as characteristic, i.e. they must be intense, have been present for a considerable time, condition the patient's behaviour, and so on.

Certain guidelines apply to the choice of potency of the remedies prescribed in these cases, even though it is commonly accepted among homoeopaths that there are no strict rules. The guidelines I follow are: firstly, to do with the simillimum – the closer the simillimum, the higher the potency and the greater the likelihood of an aggravation after the remedy; and secondly, to do with the amount of pathology in the case – if there are lesions, or problems with the excretory organs or passages, then I would begin with a low potency. However, in any given case, I would still use the potency which I considered to be correct for that particular patient at that particular time.

Case I: Oscar O., aged 22, single

Dr Detinis: Please tell me what brings you to this consultation.
Patient: I have had psychological problems since 1975. At that time I began to think I didn't have a face. My parents were always too busy to talk to so I thought I was just being silly and kept quiet about it; but in 1982 the problems got much worse – they became unbearable. At the end of March or perhaps the beginning of April of that year, I was at secondary school then, I had a kind of crisis and went to see a psychologist. I don't think he treated me properly, though. After that I saw a woman psychologist.

After a year I felt better and stopped going, but then my problems came back. I went to a church where there was another psychologist, a young woman, and she saw that I cried all the time and sent me to a hospital psychologist in Buenos Aires. Everything seemed fine and I stopped going there after a year too.

When I got engaged at the end of 1985, the problems started again and got even worse – but not because of her – they got worse and worse till I finally thought I might be homosexual. (*Screams and cries*) I can't stand it, I can't stand it any more! I'm not! I don't know why, but in 1982 I almost committed suicide. I can't go on living like this, I can't bear it, I can't stand it any more! Ten years! Ten years of pain and suffering! Do you think I enjoy being with my girlfriend and not feeling well? I can't stand it! I'm not pretending! ('Feigning sick' 48/I) . . . Ten years!

Once when I was a boy I poked my finger in a socket and got an electric shock, it made my face go contorted, it was awful. I became very aggressive – I still am. How could I want to kiss a man, attack him, kiss him . . . ! I can't stand it any more! No, I'm not homosexual, I'm not! When Rock Hudson died of Aids . . . I got scared . . . Why do I want to kiss his photograph against my own will? I don't fancy men, really I don't! I began to get scared, I don't know why. I'm sorry to be so aggressive. (*Screams and cries*)

I can't stand it any more, it's hell, living hell! Give me something, something for my mind. If it isn't treated now it could get worse (*Screams and cries*) . . . my girlfriend might leave me, I love her! . . . I can't go on any more! Look, I'll tell you something, there's no point in keeping quiet about it. In 1980 I went with a man, I thought he could help me, cure me. He told me that my problem might be sexual . . . Well, I don't know how to say this, I don't know the medical term for sleeping with someone. He took me from behind, I thought he could cure me. Yes, I did, really, I thought he could help me. It happened twice. Once with a woman; I made love to her while he took me from behind; someone was keeping lookout as this woman was married. But I don't see how that could scare me. I don't want to be homosexual! No! Not that! I want to be cured, I know I do, do you understand?

Dr Detinis: Perfectly. Do you have any other problems, Oscar?

Patient: What? Isn't that enough? It's living hell, I wanted to kill myself and my parents in 1982 . . . now you know everything. Problems? OK, I was a bit sheltered from the real world living at home. But first I want those people here to promise to keep all of this to themselves. Alright?

Dr Detinis: They are all doctors, Oscar, there's no need to worry.

Patient: Because I know someone over there, a friend of my girl-friend's, and I don't want anyone else to know about this. I was a bit sheltered because of the electric shock. I didn't have to work, I never wanted to work until I got engaged this year and had to. My parents couldn't understand why, they said I didn't have to. I saw that my problems were getting worse and worse and realised that now that I was engaged I had to go out to work . . . My girlfriend has a brother who's a policeman . . . Sometimes, I don't know, I felt like kissing him . . . I don't know why, I can't understand myself. I don't want to go from one psychologist to another, it's terrible.

Some people might think I was pretending, but I'm not, because otherwise I wouldn't be here ('Feigning sick'). I don't like acting, anyway I don't do it, at least I don't think so, I don't know about you. I don't enjoy it. If I'm not treated now I could get worse; I don't mean attacking men, although I can be really ferocious. Oh God, no! Ten years I've suffered. (*Screams and cries*) Ten years of hell! And now I'm engaged this has to happen. I can't stand it any more, I can't stand it! Please help me! My girlfriend is outside. I don't want her to leave me and I don't want to leave her. Help me! What else do you want me to tell you? I was a bit sheltered. Sometimes I don't get on with my Mum and Dad. What else do you want me to say?

Dr Detinis: Tell us how you got on with your parents, your Mum and your Dad, since you were a boy.

Patient: (*Cries*) I'm sorry I'm crying, I can't help it. I don't sleep well . . . I don't know if that's of any use to you. I don't sleep well. My girlfriend's family is against me. My parents sometimes don't under-stand me, they're a bit distant . . . they sound like they're reading from a book when they talk to me. I don't need books, I need parents. I want them to listen to me, to be my friends ... It's not that they're bad to me, they've given me a lot of nice things. But I need love and affection, I wish they would listen to me occasionally ('Forsaken feeling' (49/I)).

Perhaps if they listened to me I wouldn't go from one psychologist to another, perhaps I wouldn't be here now. I don't know what else I can tell you ... My mother is Spanish, she's quiet, doesn't have a lot to say. My father is very hardworking. Sometimes they don't understand me. She doesn't talk much; sometimes she watches soaps while I'm eating; sometimes I watch them with her. I'm sorry, I'm not effeminate or anything, but I'm scared of that. Do you know what I mean? I'm scared of that, very scared. I don't want to end up shooting myself.

My mother is a bit reserved. I think she lived through the Civil War. That's bound to have had an effect on her, she's not going to be the same as someone who had a comfortable upbringing. She left school when she was twelve. My Dad never went to school. He lived in the countryside, his father died when he was only two and he had to go out to work when he was seven. So you see my father and mother both suffered a lot and didn't want me to suffer too. I don't know what else I can tell you ...

Dr Detinis: Tell us about your character.

Patient: My character? Sometimes it seems rather vague, not like a male character at all. It always seems to spill out because I'm a very nervous sort of person. Sometimes I feel as though I could do something to you, to other people, but I don't want to! I just want you to understand that I'm suffering. Doesn't anyone realise that I'm suffering and that no one listens to me and that I sometimes get depressed? ('Forsaken feeling'). Why does this have to happen to me now that I've got a girlfriend? There must be some reason. And why do I want to attack men with strong personalities? Why? I need to know why. I need to know whether I can be cured or not!

Dr Detinis: Have you got a strong personality?

Patient: I want to attack men with strong personalities! Attack them sexually, hit them, attack them!

Dr Detinis: Is that what you do?

Patient: No, I don't! Because I've got to understand that I'm a normal person who couldn't do that. Do you see?

Dr Detinis: The impulse is there.

Patient: But it has to be eliminated, eradicated!

Dr Detinis: It stays in your mind.

Patient: Yes, but it must be eliminated.

Dr Detinis: Of course, but I have to know . . .

Patient: I don't even know where it is. Sometimes I feel like a machine that's gone out of control. And if I don't control it now, then it could get much worse. I want to have a home, get married, start a family. I don't want my children to have to go through what I've been through. What else do you want me to tell you? I want my children to be happy, because I haven't been happy. The impulse is there, but why can't I avoid it now? And if not now, then when?

Dr Detinis: Why haven't you been happy?

Patient: I've never been happy, I don't think ever. Perhaps I never tried to be happy, perhaps I thought I was happy. I don't know . . . I haven't noticed that I was ever happy except when I was with my girlfriend.

Dr Detinis: Why not?

Patient: Sometimes I don't know why. Perhaps my parents didn't understand me . . . Perhaps I didn't understand them ('Forsaken feeling'). I don't know if I'm scared of Aids or of death. Sometimes I seem scared of life more than anything else. I did tell you I thought I didn't have a face, didn't I?

Dr Detinis: Yes, perhaps you could tell me more about that.

Patient: I don't know the reason for some of these things. My girlfriend's a nurse and she might be able to say that it's schizophrenia or something like that . . .

Dr Detinis: I'm not interested in what other people think, but in what you feel right now.

Patient: I know that my opinion is valid. Why did it happen, why did I think I didn't have a face? Why?

Dr Detinis: When and in what circumstances did it occur?

Patient: In the third year of primary school. I don't know why it happened. I don't analyse myself a great deal, sometimes I find it hard to analyse myself.

Dr Detinis: Did something happen in your family, was there some upset?

Patient: No, no; it just happened, it happened and I used to masturbate and then I thought that I didn't have a face. It led on from that.

Dr Detinis: What's that about masturbation?

Patient: I masturbated on my own, I used to fantasise about someone who behaved badly and punished himself, who soiled his pants . . .

And that's what I did, that's how I punished myself. It used to excite me. I collected photos of girls and used to excite myself with them while I was masturbating ... A few years ago I saw a picture of a Jewish woman in a gas chamber – I masturbated over that ... Now I've got a girlfriend and I notice that I sometimes masturbate. Why do I do that when I've got a girlfriend? There must be some reason for it!

Dr Detinis: Doesn't it bring relief?

Patient: With her it did ... But why? I don't know why, I don't understand myself, Doctor. I don't know who I am. I want to be free of all of that. Why can't I be a normal human being, why can't I have a normal sex life, lead a normal life – why not, why can't I?

Dr Detinis: What sort of pictures did you used to masturbate with ... pictures of women?

Patient: Yes, pictures of women. Not men. Except for once – there was a picture of a sportsman and a little baby, but women excite me more. Sometimes no one seems to believe me when I say I don't want to be homosexual, as though I was pretending. But I'm not, I do want to get out of this mess ...

Dr Detinis: What we need to know is who you really are.

Patient: A boy who never knew what he wanted to do, who loves painting, who always wanted someone to love, a girl, someone who could understand him, a person who has suffered a great deal ('Forsaken feeling'). Someone whom no one believes, because he never had to work ... People used to ask me how I could suffer or have problems if I didn't have to go to work. That's what they said, I don't know why. That's when I decided I wanted to talk it over with lots of different people, people who could understand me, because that's how you learn about each other. They thought that if I didn't have to work, I couldn't suffer. Do you have to work in order to suffer? A lot of people would say so in my case.

Someone who loves painting, who loves his girlfriend; I love her very much. I say that because I'm here out of love for her. If I didn't love her then I wouldn't be here; I wouldn't go to work either. I love painting, yes I do; I don't like politicians, I hate radicals, right-wingers ... I hate lots of people, crazy people, fascists ... sometimes I seem quite hard ... I don't know if that's relevant. Is that relevant, Doctor?

Dr Detinis: Very much so.

Patient: If I was in power, I would be a hard man, I would show no mercy to my opponents, I would rise above everyone ... I hate the opposition – I'm sorry, but I do. I don't like homosexuals or prostitutes. I don't like them, I want to cure them, I want to cure myself first. I don't like priests, I don't like to see them get rich off other people, I don't like it when they keep me waiting. I can't stand red tape, I don't know if I can stand myself . . . I don't like bad actors. I'm a bit left-wing, it's true. I don't know, ever since I voted I hate politics and politicians. I don't know why. It's crazy. One thing leads on from another. If I think that I might be homosexual, what else could be wrong with me? It never goes away completely, one thing leads on from another. I like sentimental music, sentimental novels, romantic music . . . I'm a bit sentimental. Sometimes I seem to have necrophilic tendencies . . . I used to collect pictures of dead people . . . Peron, Eva Peron, Paul VI, John Paul II, though he's still alive . . . I used to collect pictures of them dressed up in different uniforms and robes . . . Then I tore them all up.

Dr Detinis: Why did you collect them?

Patient: I don't know, just to see what they looked like . . .

Dr Detinis: Why did you call yourself a necrophile?

Patient: Why? A necrophile is someone who loves dead people. You see, I never used to collect pictures of living people.

Dr Detinis: Do you know why not?

Patient: No, I never analyse myself. Sometimes I think that now I'm engaged, now's the time to pull myself together and use my brains a bit. Sometimes people seem to think that I'm some kind of moron, if you'll pardon the expression. There's a lot of aggression in me. I even had an argument with my girlfriend's brother! That's why he doesn't like me any more – he told me he wanted to help me and I felt really insulted! I do that to people sometimes, I'm afraid, if someone wants to help me I take it as an insult.

Dr Detinis: Can you tell me what happened?

Patient: I thought he was going to attack me because of the way he was talking to me. He's a tough man . . . Sometimes I don't know whether people are talking seriously or joking. It's a miracle that I actually believe in my girlfriend, because I find it so hard to believe. I've been deceived so often! I never went so far as to take drugs, but once I wanted to kill my parents and myself.

Dr Detinis: How?

Patient: Kill them with a knife and then kill myself. (*Screams and cries*) Do you think you can possibly know what I'm going through? Sometimes I think I'm like Argentina. It's as if Videla is inside me, ravaging me, destroying me. I'm rotting away! (*Screams and cries*) I can't stand it any more, nobody ever consoles me, nobody tries to help me! ('Forsaken feeling').

I cry a lot. That's another problem. I don't know what else to say. I need help because I can't stand it any more. Sometimes I feel like I'm dying or having a nervous breakdown. I'm not stupid, I've got a job washing dishes . . . I don't know if that's relevant. They said I wouldn't be able to make much of a living from painting . . . I've been working for three years. Sometimes I think about attacking someone sexually . . . a man with a beard . . . I want to know why, I want to know whether I can be cured or not. I don't want to have come here for nothing, and my girlfriend too. Give me a chance, tell me that I'm going to get better, that I'm not gay. Tell me something . . . I don't know what else to say to everybody here . . . I don't know what else to say. Tell me something!

Dr Detinis: We're here to help you, Oscar. That's why you're here.

Patient: Yes, but you're rushing me. I want you to tell me exactly what's wrong with me. Is it so bloody difficult to be normal? Am I asking too much? A normal person without mental or sexual problems? What else do you want me to say? No one ever suffered as much as I did. (*Cries*) My girlfriend is waiting outside, just think what she'll have to go through. Do you think I enjoy watching her having to put up with this? I want her to know I can be cured; I want you to tell me if I can be cured . . .

Dr Detinis: You will get much better and you will be cured, Oscar. But first we have to know more about you. You said a little while ago, 'Nobody ever consoles me'.

Patient: Nobody! I don't just want you to look at me and say, 'You wimp, you've got lots of different symptoms'. I want you to console me, forgive me. You aren't trying to console me. I don't want to be a guinea pig, I want you to say something. I'm twenty-two and I've already seen lots of psychologists!

Sometimes I think that I'm OK when I'm alone; sometimes I think I can shake off my problems, patch things up with my girlfriend's family, with my own family. Sometimes I think that being homosexual is not the problem; it's really my fear of living. Sometimes I feel like killing myself, what's the point of going on, it would be easier to be dead and in the grave . . . Wouldn't it? I'm scared of confronting life. Of course, I don't think I should repress myself, or kill myself either. Say something! I don't know, I'm sorry to go on like this but I feel that if it isn't dealt with now I'll just rot away, and I want to get married before I die. I don't want to be a homosexual or a single man, I just want to die happy. I want a happy life. Strange, eh? I always say 'die', never 'live'. It's as though it's hard to be alive, sometimes I find it hard to live with myself. What will it be like to live with someone else when I'm married?

I want to apologise to someone in the audience, I won't mention her name, it's the woman who knows my girlfriend. I'm sorry you have to listen to this. I don't like it either. Do you know what I've gone through? Sometimes I don't sleep well, I can't even eat. Do you know how awful that is? It's terrible! I like being with my girlfriend, why do I have to go through this? I'm like a Jew in a concentration camp, tortured and beaten. I don't know . . . Sometimes I think that society is like a gas chamber, it suffocates me, my fear of society. I don't want to be told how to behave, I don't want my parents to tell me how to behave, nobody! I don't know if I'm scared of all these things. I'm scared of life, because I've never known how to live . . . Sometimes I'm scared of dying. I don't know.

Dr Detinis: What else are you scared of, Oscar?
Patient: I'm scared of crossing the street, I'm scared of my girlfriend leaving me, I'm scared of talking to myself, I'm scared of talking to my girlfriend's family, talking to my family, talking to my girl-friend's brother. Talking! I'm scared of society! I'm scared of being hit, being attacked! No one was ever as scared as I am. I'm scared of the dead. How strange! I'm scared of the dead – and the living too. I'm scared of everything ('Delusions, persecuted, he is' (*Synthetic Repertory*, column 335)).

Dr Detinis: Why are you scared of dead people?
Patient: I think it's because they don't move. I'm not sure . . . Once I wanted to kiss a man in a coffin, about five years ago – I was very ill.

I'm scared I'll never be famous. I don't want my girlfriend to leave me; I don't know if that's just me being selfish. No one likes to live on their own. I'm with her because I love her and for the company, for both those reasons. How nice it is to be with the one you love. I'm scared of not being able to sleep, I'm scared that she'll leave me. I'm scared that she doesn't understand me, I'm scared that society doesn't understand me ('Forsaken feeling'). I'm scared that if I can't settle down with her then I'll never settle down with anybody.

When I was fifteen, in 1978, my father beat me because I came home late, at eight o'clock. How can you call that late? He beat me with a cane, when I was fifteen. I'm scared because my memory of it is so vivid. I'm scared. Scared of the police, of politicians . . . Scared of a lot of things ('Delusions, persecuted, he is'). Someone up there doesn't like me, look what a mess they've made of my life! I'm scared that this country is going to ruin, I'm scared that I won't be able to do anything to stop it, I'm scared I'll be silenced.

I'm scared of so many things. I'm even scared of crossing the street because in about 1974 I was knocked down by a car; the driver had his arm in plaster. I didn't have a girlfriend then. I was injured. And in 1982 when I was leaving my painting class, I was knocked down by another car. And this year when I went to the cinema with my girl-friend's family, I just missed being knocked down again.

I'm scared of death. Sometimes I think I'm lying in a coffin, I feel as if I'm suffocating and want to get out. I'm scared of being like that man in the picture; scared of being dead. I'm scared, scared! I don't know why I'm scared of suffocating if I was lying in a coffin, because you can't suffocate when you're dead. I'm scared of being cremated. I'm scared of life, I'm scared of death. I'm scared of not being able to love properly, I'm scared of wanting to be in a relationship, I'm scared. Lots of things. I'm scared of wanting to attack you, them. I'm scared, scared that you might beat me and call the police. I don't want to die in prison. I don't want to be locked up in a mental home.

Dr Detinis: I should like to ask you a few questions.
Patient: Yes, ask me anything you like! All I want is to be cured. I'll tell you everything, everything!

Dr Detinis: How does the weather affect you, Oscar?
Patient: The weather? My hands get sweaty . . . When I have those problems with my girlfriend's brother, I sweat a bit more. I'm sweat-ing right now. I sweat when it's hot and I sweated when I thought I didn't have a face, it felt sort of exciting. I sweat a lot. When I say something stupid I sweat even more. I sweat when it's hot, more when I get sexually aroused, that's when I sweat most.

Dr Detinis: Where do you sweat most?
Patient: My hands . . . All over my body, my back . . .

Dr Detinis: And what is the sweat like?
Patient: Sometimes it's pretty unbearable, it's a male smell! I'm a man, not a . . .

Dr Detinis: Where is this strong smell?
Patient: Under the armpits. And when I'm making love I can some-times smell my own strong smell . . . I sweat a lot when I'm aroused.

128

Case I: Oscar O., aged 22, single

Dr Detinis: Is the sweat greasy or runny?

Patient: Runny. But my face is sometimes greasy. And my feet sweat a lot. Sometimes I get an impulse to embrace you ('Embraces everyone'). . . . but I think you'd try and stop me. Sometimes I think people would say I was gay if I wanted to embrace someone, embrace a man, just in a friendly way. They wouldn't like it if I tried to embrace a girl either. It makes me sweat when I think that.

Dr Detinis: What kind of food do you like?

Patient: I don't like milk.

Dr Detinis: Sweet things?

Patient: Yes, but I'm also scared of putting on weight. I'm scared of absolutely everything.

Dr Detinis: Do you like salt?

Patient: I don't like very salty things.

Dr Detinis: Fruit?

Patient: Yes, all kinds of fruit. Avocados, apples, I like them all.

Dr Detinis: Do you prefer fruit to other kinds of food?

Patient: No, not particularly.

Dr Detinis: Do you like spicy things?

Patient: Yes, the spicy meat stews that my Mum makes, they're fantastic! Stews, salty things . . .

Dr Detinis: Vinegar and lemons?

Patient: Yes, everything like that. I can't drink alcohol though.

Dr Detinis: Why not?

Patient: Because I'm on medication. I'm taking Serenace and Lorazepam – 2mg of Lorazepam and five drops of Serenace. If I drank wine I'd probably explode. I don't smoke either. I'm scared of lung cancer too.

Dr Detinis: Just cancer?

Patient: Cancer and other horrible diseases. I don't know what else.

Dr Detinis: Do you have a recurring dream, Oscar?

Patient: I dream a lot, mostly when I'm with my girlfriend; but I never have the same dream twice. Once I dreamt that I was sleeping with my girlfriend – her parents don't like us sleeping together – and I dreamt that they came and woke me up and were nice to me. It seemed so real but in real life it's not like that! I used to dream that I said something to my girlfriend on the phone, something that wasn't true, and she shouted down the phone at me and then I woke up and it wasn't really true. I often dream when I'm with my girlfriend . . .

Dr Detinis: Well . . .

Patient: Wait! Sometimes I dream that I will rule a country and then my Dad says, 'Rule this country?' Don't be daft!' ('Delusions, great person, is' (26/II)).

Dr Detinis: Oscar . . .

Patient: Wait! There's another dream. I dream that I go and see my old psychologist and he says, 'So you left me and went to another psychologist, did you?' I dream about being taken to a concentration camp with the Jews, going to the gas chamber in a train and being completely naked . . .

Dr Detinis: Do you mind if my colleagues ask you a few questions?

Patient: Anything, anything. I know it's all for my own good.

QUESTIONS FROM THE FLOOR

Question: Oscar, when you say something and someone contradicts you, how do you react?

Patient: When I say something and someone contradicts me? I don't like to be contradicted. Once my girlfriend's brother said something – according to my girlfriend he was trying to help me – and I took it as an insult, I just sneered at him! Sometimes I want to criticise, be a typical Nazi. Sometimes it makes me want to cry.

Question: Oscar, were you born in Argentina?

Patient: Yes, in Lanus, in 1963.

Question: Could I ask you why you have what sounds like a foreign accent?

Patient: Yes, I'll tell you why: that's because I put my finger in a socket when I was a little baby, I got an electric shock right through my body and that's what made me aggressive. It also gave me speech problems and that's why I've got a funny accent. People say I sound like a German Jew.

Question: Oscar, what is it about the Nazis and the Jews that makes you talk about them all the time?

Patient: Alright, I'll tell you. It was the way in which the Nazis killed people. And the fact that they killed young women. The crazy way in which they killed the Jews; so cruel and brutal. That's what it is – that image of the violence.

And the Jews because they were persecuted by everyone, they're still persecuted now. They were whipped and beaten by everyone. Do you know that I have suffered a great deal and sometimes identify myself with the Jews? I've suffered as much as they have; I've been whipped and beaten by everyone. The Peronists threw me out of their party . . . my girlfriend's family is against me, sometimes my own family is. The Jews were as persecuted as I am. That's what it is. We're the same ('Delusions, persecuted, he is'). Sometimes I feel like a Jewish refugee.

Question: By whom do you feel persecuted, Oscar?
Patient: Society! This sexist, corrupt, murderous, criminal society . . . I feel persecuted because they don't understand me. I feel persecuted by my girlfriend's family. If I do or say anything I feel persecuted. By society in general. I don't know whether society is to blame, or me. I don't know . . . I feel so persecuted . . . By the radicals . . .

Question: And how exactly do you feel when you feel persecuted?
Patient: I can't say what I feel like! Sometimes I feel like I want to say, 'The police are corrupt because they never pay their fare when they go on the bus', but I don't because I'm scared that I'd get beaten up. I'm scared, very scared.

Question: You never say anything?
Patient: No, because no one ever listens to me. No one wants to listen to me! Sometimes I feel very bad because I'm scared that if I say something to my girlfriend, she might leave me; if I say something to my girlfriend's family they'll make her leave me. Or I'm scared . . . of being rejected by society. Of no one ever saying, 'No, Oscar, we're not going to persecute you . . .' But I am persecuted! I'm very scared.

Question: When was the worst time in your life, Oscar?
Patient: When I got the electric shock. And in December 1977, my aunt committed suicide. I didn't know the truth until 1982. The other time was when I had the mental attack. (*Cries*) In March 1981 I had a very strong attack and wanted to kill myself. I couldn't even say: 'This is my family'. That was the worst time of my life. Actually the worst time of my life was when I wanted to say things I didn't mean to my girlfriend. I wanted to say I didn't love her when really I did. Those were the worst times of my life.

Question: How did you want to kill yourself, Oscar?
Patient: I wanted to kill myself with a knife, or take an overdose of pills, or shoot myself. I'm a coward, I'm very scared of dying. I don't know if that means I want to live. I'm crying because I want to live. . . . (*Screams and cries*) I want to live! I want to live! More than ever

131

now that I'm engaged. I want you to listen to me, I don't want you to go away! I want you to listen to me, to help me! I can't take it any more. I have to scream so society will hear me and say, 'Here's Oscar, let's help him!'

I'm so scared of taking a knife and killing my parents! . . . Other worst times are when people think that I'm not really crying, that I'm just pretending to cry – I hate that ('Feigning sick'). But I'm powerless . . . I'm also scared of Down's syndrome. I would like to help all homosexuals and everyone with Down's syndrome . . . if I had the money . . .

COMMENTARY

Oscar's case is a most unusual one. Before I go into it, I should like to make a few general points about psychiatric cases, or cases in which mental symptoms are present to such a degree.

The question we must ask ourselves is this: If we regard the psychiatric illness as an organic entity, which symptoms should we take into account?

Psychiatric symptoms may be common ones that should be disregarded. They may also have significance as homoeopathic symptoms when they have modalities or when they express the individual's character, provided of course that the corresponding symptom exists in the materia medica.

As is the case with other mental symptoms, psychiatric symptoms are, in general, neither more nor less than an exaggeration. All human beings have characteristics which form their psychological profile. Symptoms cannot be drawn from these, for they are normal characteristics; but when they are exaggerated, weakened or deformed they become homoeopathic symptoms in the repertory and in the materia medica. These symptoms are an expression of a disturbance in the vital force, so they are pathological by definition. There is no essential difference between normal characteristics and the symptoms in the repertory, except that, as we see in the present case, the symptoms appear with greater force and create a sort of caricature of the person.

Oscar has characteristics which could be considered from a psychiatric point of view, but they are also homoeopathic symptoms which have their counterpart in the materia medica. Despite the psychiatric pathology evident in Oscar, I do not need to adopt a psychiatric approach (although I can determine whether the particular disorder he is suffering from is schizophrenia or hysteria). If we can arrive at a clear understanding of Oscar's problem we should be able to find the remedy without too much difficulty.

What then is he suffering from? The fundamental symptom, which cannot be ignored, is 'Forsaken feeling' (49/I). He expressed this in every possible way, particularly when talking of his relationship with his parents. Much of his behaviour is conditioned by a feeling of being abandoned. He said, 'My parents don't understand me . . . they sound like books when they talk to me. They gave me lots of nice things, but I want them to listen to me, I need love and affection . . . Perhaps if they listened to me I wouldn't go from one psychologist to another.' All of this shows clearly what he is suffering from. He goes to see psychologists because he has not received enough affection, because no one pays any attention or listens to him. He said, 'Doesn't anyone realise that I'm suffering and that no one ever listens to me?' He fears that his girlfriend will leave him, and tells us that no one consoles him. We cannot ignore this symptom – the remedy we choose must be in this rubric.

There are other important symptoms, as for example 'Feigning sick' (48/I) which appeared right at the beginning of the consultation. At one point he was crying but also looking at me to see if I was watching him. He has a tendency to feign and to take people in – he said it in so many words: 'I'm not pretending, but you don't believe me', and '. . . anyway, I'm not acting'. In such circumstances we must take the patient's words to mean the opposite of what they say; we cannot take them at face value. I was in no way moved to sympathise with his suffering, simply because he was feigning. This symptom was clearly expressed on several occasions and is one of the characteristics of his illness. He has a tendency to exaggerate the problems he is suffering from; his psychiatric condition contains some elements of hysteria.

Another symptom is 'Delusions, persecuted, he is' (*Synthetic Repertory*, column 335). He is scared of the police: 'I'm scared that I'd get beaten up'. When someone tries to help him, as his girlfriend's brother did, he feels they are trying to attack him: 'I'm scared of being hit, being attacked'. This is a persecution mania.

A fourth symptom is 'Delusions, great person, is' (26/II). He fears he will never be famous. He has delusions of grandeur and feels that he is more important than everyone else: 'I dream that I will rule the country'. He looks down on people in power because they are stupid and he is scared they may exercise their power over him.

Then there is his great fear of homosexuality, which does not feature in the repertory. He must have strong tendencies towards

Case Studies

homosexuality in order to be struggling against it with such force. There are other symptoms which cannot be found in the materia medica, such as necrophilia. Besides collecting photos of Peron and Paul IV, he said that five years ago he kissed a dead man, and it seems quite clear that his feelings were other than those of a man paying last respects. This is necrophilia, a psychiatric condition which may involve sexual acts with dead bodies.

Oscar also has the characteristic symptom of wanting to embrace everyone, which appears in *MacRepertory*.

REPERTORISATION

'Forsaken feeling' (49/I)
'Feigning sick' (48/I)
'Delusions, persecuted, he is' (*Synthetic Repertory*, column 335)
'Embraces everyone' (*MacRepertory*)
'Delusions, great person, is' (26/II)

Prescription: Veratrum Album 1M.

The emotional symptoms, which correspond to what Kent called the symptoms of the will, are the ones that lie deepest. In general, only Phosphorus and Pulsatilla cover more of them than Veratrum Album (although this is not the case with Oscar). Veratrum is in fact a great polychrest, with many other applications beyond the domain of psychiatry.

FOLLOW-UP

(*Seven months after the first prescription*)

Patient: I'm feeling better, I'm not so crazy as I was before. I'm much calmer. I worry that people won't believe me when I say this. I'm not aggressive and I don't have my old headaches. I don't have homosexual fantasies any more and I don't have the desire to collect photos of important men . . . now if they were women instead! (*Laughs jokingly*) I don't imagine that people are about to attack me. What bothers me now is that my parents don't have any time for me. I've been working for the Diabetics Association, selling tickets.

Prescription. Placebo.

Case II: Marta, aged 42, married, two daughters

Dr Detinis: Please tell me what you would like to discuss.
Patient: I've got a problem with my spine, I've had two operations . . .
Shall I tell you when my problem started? Well, it all started after my
first child was born. I went to see a doctor . . . I had a pain in my waist,
I went to see an orthopaedic surgeon and he told me that I had lumbago
caused by herniation of an intervertebral disc. They made me wear a
plaster corset and I had it on for six and a half weeks. I didn't have any
neurological problems, I just had lumbar pains. Then they took it off. I
was alright for a while and then a year later I twisted my spine and they
sent me back to have another plaster corset fitted, but then I began to
have neurological problems in my left leg. They did a myelogram and
it showed that I had pressure on the fourth lumbar root.

The corset didn't help at all, I couldn't walk any more, and when
they took it off I was more twisted than ever, and they were going to
operate on me – despite the risk involved – and a friend took me to a
very good orthopaedic surgeon, who is now dead, and he managed to
put the disc back in place with chiropractic, external manipulations. He
told me that the fibrous ring was ruptured; he gave me injections in my
hip, not steroids, but something else.

After the first session I could stand up straight again, I felt so much
better: he continued treating me three times a week for a month and
after six months the pain in my leg had completely gone and I was fine,
completely better. But when I had my second child seven years later I
slipped a disc again and I went back to him for more treatment and I
did really well, but after that I had to go back to him more and more
frequently. I'd feel pain every time I moved my back. I would go back
to the chiropractor and he'd give me a massage . . . nothing violent,
you understand, no sharp cracks or anything, he would just gently
traction my spine with the palms of his hands until he could feel things
moving . . . I never heard anything moving inside, and it never hurt
me – on the contrary, it felt really comfortable. I used to talk to him a
lot, ask him to tell me what he was doing to me. He'd say, 'It's gone
back into place a bit more now'. The problem was my vertebrae kept
coming out of place, and what he did was put them back, and then I'd
feel so much better.

In 1983 my daughter had an operation on her throat, and seven hours
later she started losing blood and she cried for me, 'Mummy, Mummy,
Mummy!' so of course I bent down and picked her up, and a few days

135

later I had the lumbago back again ('Speech, repeats same thing', *Synthetic Repertory*, column 943).

Meanwhile the doctor had died, and things began to get very complicated. I could move about alright, but I began to get a burning sensation at the base of my spine, in my buttocks, and from the knees up to the thighs, it was itching and itching and itching, it was driving me mad with the itching! ('Speech, repeats'). This went on for eight months! The orthopaedic surgeons said there was nothing wrong with me, but it was driving me mad! I had no lumbago, just this itching which spread all over my back, with perspiration all over my back. I would wake up at night completely drenched in sweat with my head and whole body burning. It got to the point where my whole body was burning.

Then I was taken to see a Japanese man, and he told me to lie on the couch – he'd already seen the X-rays – so he told me to lie on the couch, and he pressed his heel into my lower back. This was my first experience of violent chiropractic treatment; I didn't feel any pain but I felt that all my bones . . . he told me to lie on my side and crack! I felt it down my whole spine. He said, 'You take lots of vitamins, lady, lots of vitamins.' He gave me a huge supply of vitamin supplements to take away with me.

I began to put on weight and I got better and better and better ('Speech, repeats'). Then about a week later my groin started to get very painful, like a throbbing nerve pain. I felt I had more energy a few days later, I could feel the circulation in my legs was better because I could feel them burning and then suddenly my feet became cold; I could feel the blood coming back into them, and the itching stopped. I began to feel something like scar tissue growing inside my buttocks, like something was forming a scar inside me; but then after three months of this the pain came back, just pain, pain, and more pain ('Speech, repeats'). They did some CT scans on me, they did a myelogram and then they took me to see this man who'd given me the chiropractic before. The myelogram showed that I had chronic nerve damage at L4 and L5, sensory nerve damage, which had shown up on the myelogram, and that's why I was getting the itching sensations, and the CT scan showed that between the fourth and fifth vertebrae the disc space had narrowed and there was a growth at the left-hand side of the vertebrae.

Then I got these crawling sensations in my legs like pins and needles and the neurosurgeon . . . Oh, I forgot, he also told me that there was a problem with my intervertebral discs at L4 and L5, and after radiological examination they discovered that I had intervertebral lesions at L4 and L3 as well. I went in for an operation to stretch the vertebral column and to let them have a closer look a the intervertebral discs. After the operation the neurosurgeon explained what was wrong . . . apparently I had compression of the spinal cord at L4 and L5, and he had removed the protruding part of the intervertebral disc, leaving me half a disc on each side, and he had also stretched the vertebral column at L4, L5 and part of L3. Five days after the operation I began to feel very frightened. I told the surgeon and he said 'Why?'. 'Because I'm getting cramps all up my legs from my knees to my groin, all my muscles are cramping up and my groin is very painful, there's pain all around my pelvis', I said.

Months went by, all they prescribed for me were vitamins, but they didn't help. I felt worse and worse, worse and worse ('Speech, repeats'). They did another CT scan and discovered that I had an acute protrusion of an intervertebral disc at L3, it was as round as a ball. It showed up on the scan as round as a ball, protruding out of the column. Then, not satisfied with that, they did another myelogram and the neurosurgeon diagnosed that I had a post-surgical cyst – that's what he said it was, a post-surgical cyst. So I went in for another operation, but he couldn't find the cyst, or the protruding disc. Then he tells me that I haven't got an intervertebral disc, because he couldn't find it. And all he could do was stretch more of the spinal column, from L2 to the sacrum.

It's seventeen months since I was operated on and my symptoms are getting worse – I've still got the pain in my groin but all they can do is take more myelograms and tell me that the nerves aren't damaged. I get these pulling sensations down there but they tell me there's no damage to the motor nerves which go from the knees to the ankle, meanwhile I'm still getting the pulling sensations . . . and it turns out there is some damage to the sensory nerves . . . I get these crawling sensations . . . the muscles from my knee to my groin are just wasting away. He told me that he'd stretched my vertebral column to make more room for the nerve but that that couldn't be the cause of the pain. He did another CT scan and the protrusion didn't show up, it didn't show up on the CT scan ('Speech, repeats'). And now they say they don't want to do any more tests on me because I've been through so much.

But I'm still in pain after all these months, I still get the crawling sensations up and down my spine, and the sweating . . . I sometimes feel a cold sweat along my spine, it's like a burning feeling; and I wake up at night and even my head feels like it's burning; and if I get up and walk about my vision comes over all blurred and I get a feeling of pressure at the sides of my head . . . it's not a dizzy feeling, I don't ever faint or anything like that, but I get such a pain in my back that if I lean over my back feels so bruised and battered, it's even worse if I touch it, and I get this itching in my legs, if I move them in a certain way, they start to itch and itch and itch, ('Speech, repeats'), it spreads all over my genitals, all over my legs, it's terrible, and the pain in my groin is constantly there.

I'm not on any medication now, I've tried the lot and nothing has done any good. When I get the itching sensation now I also get problems with my circulation, I get these dark patches like bruises on my legs that last a few days. First they're yellow, then they turn black, and then they go, and they always come up in the same place. When the itching is really, really bad I take Lorazepam and that helps a bit. My whole body feels bruised and battered, absolutely exhausted, my hands and feet get so cold, so cold that they feel burning hot; if you felt my back you'd notice it was completely covered in sweat, especially up and down the spine.

Dr Detinis: And do you have any symptoms other than those related to your spine?

Patient: Well I don't know what symptoms you mean. I'm completely out of sorts. There is something . . . I'll tell you about it. A year ago when I was examining myself like this I discovered a lump. They did an ultrasound scan and I've got two fibromas and a cyst in the left ovary, it was very inflamed. They did a scan and at three o'clock that same night it swelled up because of the inflammation and the fluids.

They admitted me to the hospital, put me on a drip, it went away and I was discharged after two weeks without having been diagnosed. My gynaecologist gave me medication and told me to keep an eye on the fibromas, but what with the problem with my spine, I didn't really think it was that important because my periods are normal . . .

Dr Detinis: What are your periods like?

Patient: The one this month was normal, the month before it was a week early, but it was quite light.

Dr Detinis: What were they like before?

Patient: Normal, they came every twenty-eight days and lasted for six days.

Dr Detinis: Have you ever noticed any changes before, during or after menstruation?

Patient: No.

Dr Detinis: Any changes in your character?

Patient: No. On the whole I don't know how I manage to bear it so well, because my problem is quite . . . sometimes I don't even have the strength in my legs to go up the stairs . . .

Dr Detinis: Tell me something about yourself.

Patient: Do you mean about this problem . . . ?

Dr Detinis: No, just about yourself.

Patient: I'm a teacher . . . Well, actually now I'm retired, because three years ago I was on sick leave and when the orthopaedic surgeons saw my spine they made me retire. I'm qualified to teach moderately mentally handicapped people, as well as blind and deaf people.

Dr Detinis: What took you into that?

Patient: It's something I like very much.

Dr Detinis: How did you start?

Patient: Well, I was always interested in kids with problems; when I first went into it my parents didn't approve . . . at least my mother didn't, my father encouraged me. So I went on as many courses as I could in order to become better trained. I'm basically qualified to work with handicapped children and with blind and deaf people. I was very sad to have to give it all up and I think that when I get better I'd like to go back into it. I really like it.

Dr Detinis: What else can you tell us?

Patient: I'm very fond of children with problems and I've always worked in deprived areas; that adds a whole new dimension to a teacher's job, because often you have to go out looking for children that don't turn up to school, and at that point you're more like a social worker than a teacher . . . It's all very interesting. And well, I've always been very sure of myself, and very . . . ('Positiveness' (69/II)) . . . I don't know if it was because I'm used to working with children . . . and I've always worked with boys more than with girls; I've also worked with handicapped men. I've always got on very well with my daughters, especially the older one. I take an interest in what they do at school . . . when they do work in groups they always ask me to help them drawing pictures or things like that . . . as it's something I'm good at . . . Well, what else can I say – I'm very happy, I'm happily married . . .

Dr Detinis: You get on well with your husband?

Patient: Yes, very well.

Dr Detinis: What else?

Patient: I've always had lots of self-confidence, I don't know if I said that ('Positiveness').

Dr Detinis: What makes you say that?

Patient: Well, I've always felt very happy about what I did. Once I got married I had to make lots of sacrifices and be very well organised if I wanted to get anything done. I was very active and managed to do lots of things every day, I never forgot anything, and I was very busy and successful. I held two teaching posts, one in the city and one outside, and I always managed to make enough time for everything and I was involved in lots of different things, with my daughters, my husband, with my school ('Industrious' (56/I)).

I didn't have much time for a social life, though, because at weekends we'd rather be with the children and do something with them . . . go to the circus, or the cinema or a show . . . always the four of us together. So I didn't have a social life in the sense of just going out with my husband . . . when we go out it's always the four of us together.

My husband's job takes him away from home a lot . . . I think that's what gives me so much confidence with children, because I've always had to take over from my husband. If ever one of my daughters had a problem while he was away on business, we would always pretend to 'ask Daddy', and I would play the head of the family. So you see, I've always tried to do the best I could. That's what I meant when I said I've always been very sure of myself, I know I can always be the perfect mother when my husband isn't there! But now that I'm not very well it's psychologically much harder . . . that's what worries me most as far as my girls are concerned.

Dr Detinis: In what sense?

Patient: Well of course because I can't . . . there I am in bed all the time and I have to ask them to do all the things that I should . . . they really shouldn't have to . . . The other day my youngest went to a birthday party and the eldest had to go and pick her up.

Dr Detinis: What were you like as a girl?

Patient: According to my mother I was an angel, I was always very good – she would give me my dummy and I would quietly sit in my cot. We had an elderly relative who was very ill for a long time and so she left me in my cot or gave me some toys to play with and I was . . . fantastic!

Dr Detinis: Why do you say 'fantastic'?

Patient: Because both my parents were amazing people; they were both Asians. My father was very strict with us but also very kind and affectionate. I had one brother and one sister, my brother died seven years ago . . . I was Daddy's favourite daughter. I get on well with my mother too. Daddy died too.

Dr Detinis: What did your brother die of?

Patient: A heart attack. My sister's a dentist, six years younger than me. I always got on extremely well with my brother. I didn't get on so well with my sister because of the age gap. There was a bit of a character clash too; she was highly-strung, a very delicate child, she used to cry all the time. When she got married, my mother wasn't very well, and my father had died a year before – my sister didn't get on very well with my mother either – I organised everything. I spent three months making all the arrangements for a wedding with five hundred guests, I did everything but make the dress.

Dr Detinis: Hand on heart, how do you really feel about your sister?

Patient: I love her very much; I don't get on too well with her but I love her very much.

Dr Detinis: Don't you have any other feelings towards her, towards your parents?

Patient: No.

Dr Detinis: Jealousy?

Patient: Goodness, no! I'm not a jealous person.

Dr Detinis: What was the biggest trauma in your life?

Patient: The death of my brother, that was a great blow.

Dr Detinis: Did you find that hard to get over?

Patient: I did. My mother couldn't get over it, and a year later she had a heart attack herself. She's much better now, she took my father's death very well. Daddy had heart trouble too, so by then . . . When I was in hospital last year, she got very upset and had a second heart attack. She's much better now, but not completely because it affected the other side, but she can walk again now.

Dr Detinis: What else can you tell me about your character? Something that isn't perhaps quite so 'perfect'?

Patient: Oh, you'd have to ask my husband!

Dr Detinis: What would your husband say?

Patient: He'd say that when I believe something there's no one in the world who can make me change my mind. That I've got lots of self-confidence. He's got complete confidence in me ('Positiveness').

Dr Detinis: What else would your husband say?

Patient: I don't know, that I'm an excellent mother, an excellent wife, that when there's something to do I get on with it, that I've helped him a great deal in everything . . . The other day I told him, 'Right, I'm determined to get better, and the day I recover I'll start a school here, or I'll go back to work ('Positiveness'). And then he said, 'I've got to hand it to you, you really mean it, don't you! I know you will, if it's the last thing you do!' And then I knew that I was going to get better.

Dr Detinis: Are you an optimist?

Patient: With regard to myself, yes.

Dr Detinis: And with regard to other things?

Patient: Yes, I'm optimistic about everything. If I'm not light-hearted, people think there's something wrong with me because I'm all serious and quiet, but it's just that I'm deep in thought.

Dr Detinis: When they see you like that do they worry?

Patient: Yes, they think I'm in a bad mood.

Dr Detinis: Are you a serious, reserved sort of person?

Patient: Yes, I am, I don't often laugh. There are times when I laugh, when I crack jokes and play the fool, but on the whole I'm an introvert.

Dr Detinis: One wouldn't think so, you seem quite the opposite.

Patient: Maybe, but I am introverted, that's why I said I sometimes become serious. It's like that with my friends too, they tell me that it takes a long time to get to know me well. Because if I don't like something I don't keep quiet about it, I come right out with it.

Dr Detinis: You don't keep quiet?

Patient: No, I think it over, and when I say something it's because I'm quite sure of what I'm saying.

Dr Detinis: Don't you just chat with your friends?

Patient: Oh, yes, I do, but sometimes they notice that I'm serious and then they ask me what's the matter with me.

Dr Detinis: Do you tell them about your problems?

Patient: Yes I do, but just my closest friends . . . I could count them on the fingers of one hand.

Dr Detinis: Why do you say that?

Patient: Because real friends have to be all-round friends, don't you think? You can't have one kind for work and one for play . . . you have to cover both.

Dr Detinis: And how do you get on with your friends?

Patient: Very well.

Dr Detinis: Do you see much of them?

Patient: Oh, yes. My closest friend is a psychologist. She's my daughter's godmother, and she was a witness at my wedding, so ... she's the one I talk to most, almost every day.

Dr Detinis: Do you need to see them?

Patient: They call me to see how I am, whom I've seen, and since I'm not well, I have to make an effort, I can't be ... They help me like that and sometimes when I feel really bad they give me a bit of therapy, on the phone though!

Dr Detinis: When you're not well do you need to communicate, does it make you feel better to phone them?

Patient: Sometimes yes, but sometimes I feel so bad that ...

Dr Detinis: When you feel depressed ... ?

Patient: That's one thing I never am, I never get depressed. I'm always solid as a rock, but at the moment my problem does tend to rule my life because it's obviously pretty serious ... I wanted to cry because I said to myself, 'Why do I always have to be so self-confident?' Right now I could do with some support. Not psychological support, just something to give me a bit of a fillip. I think I know what it is, and I'm looking for it, but I also need a ... because I've always been so sure of what I've done, you see. My father always used to say, 'If it's alright by Marta then it's alright by me.'

Dr Detinis: Why did your father say that?

Patient: Because I always used to think things through before doing them, we used to weigh up the pros and cons together ...

Dr Detinis: Would your daughters say you had any shortcomings?

Patient: My daughters ...

Dr Detinis: Have they ever said anything to you?

Patient: My eldest daughter is worried, very worried about me, and ever since she was small people have said that they thought we were sisters ('Coquettish, too much', *Synthetic Repertory*, column 187).

Dr Detinis: Why is that?

Patient: Well naturally I was much slimmer, and I've never looked my age. Now I think, well, I don't know, but if you're overweight you always ... And her friends ... I remember we were once at a birthday party and someone said to my daughter – that must have been about six years ago - someone said, 'You're Mummy's so pretty!' So I would have thought that my daughter ... the eldest one – the other one's very wilful – the eldest is very well-adjusted and self-confident, but the little one is rather . . . she's a good girl though she's very wilful. I do have problems with her, but for six years now, ever since she was at nursery school, I've been practically confined to bed and as I said I can't . . .

Dr Detinis: Do you get upset easily?

Patient: Yes.

Dr Detinis: What things upset you?

Patient: I'm upset now, talking about this.

Dr Detinis: What else do you get upset by?

Patient: Talking about my brother and talking about my daughters when I can't . . . when I can't do what any mother . . . It's awful to have a mother who's ill. And however much I'd like to overcome it by sheer willpower it's impossible, because when you have a disability problem . . . They look after me so well. 'Where are you going, Mummy?' the little one asked, and the eldest one said, 'When are you coming back . . .?'

Dr Detinis: Are you an orderly and tidy person?

Patient: Hah, incredibly.

Dr Detinis: What's that, why did you say 'incredibly'?

Patient: Well, I told you before that I used to do six or seven different things every . . . And I'm very particular with my children's things – I don't like to see them left lying around . . .

Dr Detinis: You're tidy with the children's things?

Patient: Of course, I always make sure that their clothes and school things are in their proper place . . .

Dr Detinis: Would you say you are neat and tidy?

Patient: Yes, I am . . .

Dr Detinis: Respectful?

Patient: Yes, I respect their things and their tastes . . . They're great pals with their Mum, their friends come along and say, 'I want to talk to your Mummy'. I'm used to being with children and cheering them up, I've done it for so long. That's what I said to the doctor who told me I had to retire. He asked me why I was crying and I said to him, 'Because you're making me give up not just one but two different jobs.'

Dr Detinis: Just to return for a moment to the subject of tidiness, would say you're meticulous?

Patient: I used to be, though I'm less like that now.

Dr Detinis: Were you a bit fanatical about order?

Patient: No, I don't think so . . . If you were to ask my husband he would say I was. I always liked everything to be in its place, but I never shouted at him to go and tidy away his clothes . . . That's how it is, really. He isn't terribly tidy but . . . I was always very tidy, but it never got to the point where I complained about things being left lying around. No, I would go and pick them up, I did it . . .

Dr Detinis: Are you conscientious, does everything have to be just right?

Patient: Yes, I always have been, everything had to be perfect when I was choosing things for the house . . . perhaps not with regard to . . . I used to love wearing necklaces, now I don't any more . . . ('Coquettish').

Dr Detinis: Why not?

Patient: Because things are different now.

Dr Detinis: But you used to wear necklaces . . . ?

Patient: Yes, yes, yes, and rings and things . . .

Dr Detinis: Do you like that sort of thing?

Patient: Oh, yes!

Dr Detinis: Are you afraid of anything?

Patient: No.

Dr Detinis: Absolutely nothing?

Patient: Well, with everything that's happened to me I'm a bit scared of . . . not of dying, I was never scared of death, but of becoming an invalid.

Dr Detinis: Are you scared of heights, or of enclosed spaces . . . ?

Patient: I don't like them, I can't breathe.

Dr Detinis: At what sort of height?

Patient: I never fly, I've only ever been in a plane once . . . and I can't look out of an eighth floor window . . .

Dr Detinis: What about a first floor window?

Patient: I can now, but once I thought I was going to . . . Hah! I'm scared of heights . . . I used to climb up trees, and one day my husband came along and said, 'What on earth are you doing up there?' and there I was clutching on to the top of a pine tree!'

Dr Detinis: Are you scared of being alone?

Patient: No.

Dr Detinis: Scared of storms . . . ?

Patient: Not a bit!

Dr Detinis: Of thieves, dogs?
Patient: No.

Dr Detinis: Scared if you see an accident, blood?
Patient: No!

Dr Detinis: It doesn't affect you?
Patient: No.

Dr Detinis: How did you feel when you had to take exams or before an important occasion?
Patient: You sound just like a psychoanalyst! You asked me if I'm ever scared; well, they wanted me to undergo a seven-hour operation to fix the vertebrae ... Everyone else was against it, but I said that I'd go through with it, despite the risk, I really wasn't scared. I said I wanted to carry on until I got better, no matter what. I'm not scared of operations, they don't frighten me at all. As long as I'm well, I'm not scared. That's fairly convincing proof, don't you think?

Dr Detinis: Would you say you were vindictive?
Patient: Yes. You mean being angry and remembering what someone did to you?

Dr Detinis: Yes.
Patient: If I get hold of that surgeon I'll kill him!

Dr Detinis: What?
Patient: What do you think? He's the one who wrecked my whole life, and my family's too, everything! I'll make him pay for it! ('Malicious' (63/II)).

Dr Detinis: How does the weather affect you?
Patient: The weather? Do you mean whether it's hot or cold? I don't like Cordoba in the summer because it's so close.

Dr Detinis: What else?
Patient: I prefer the cold.

Dr Detinis: What does the heat do to you?
Patient: I can't bear the heat, I sweat so much anyway at the moment ... but we've got a swimming pool and everyone comes and uses it and that's nice.

Dr Detinis: And different kinds of weather? How do they affect you mentally and physically; what happens to you during a thunderstorm, or when it's windy, or humid, when you're in the sun?

Patient: Ah! I love to sunbathe; I like to have a nice tan ('Coquettish'). And the cold, well, there's always the heating.

Dr Detinis: Does any particular type of clothing bother you?

Patient: No, no – you mean do I dislike having wool against my skin or anything like that? No, no.

Dr Detinis: Does clothing on any particular part of your body bother you?

Patient: Now, yes.

Dr Detinis: What about before?

Patient: No, never.

Dr Detinis: Bodices, belts, stockings, collars . . .

Patient: No, but I couldn't wear tight trousers because they stopped my circulation. That was when I was being treated by my doctor.

Dr Detinis: And before the problems with your health?

Patient: No.

Dr Detinis: On what part of your body do you sweat?

Patient: I never sweat.

Dr Detinis: But surely you sweat a little, don't you, when you exert yourself?

Patient: Never, doctor.

Dr Detinis: Under the armpits, below your breasts, on your neck, your head, your feet . . .

Patient: I've never sweated.

Dr Detinis: Never, ever? Not until you had these problems?

Patient: Never. ('Skin, inactivity' (1326/II)).

Dr Detinis: What sort of food do you like?

Patient: I like everything except for rice pudding, absolutely everything.

Dr Detinis: And milk by itself?

Patient: Yes, I like it that too.

Dr Detinis: Sweet things?

Patient: I like them all.

Dr Detinis: Lemons, vinegar?

Patient: Those too.

Dr Detinis: Animal fat?

Patient: Yes, there's lots of that in Asian cooking, lots of lard, lots of fat . . . I like everything, except for rice pudding.

Dr Detinis: And is there something that you particularly like, that you can't resist?

Patient: No, not really.

Dr Detinis: How hot do you like your tea and coffee?

Patient: Tepid, I don't like them too hot.

Dr Detinis: How well did you used to sleep?

Patient: I slept very little.

Dr Detinis: And did you wake up easily in the mornings?

Patient: Yes, right away . . .

Dr Detinis: Did you sleep very little because you were so busy?

Patient: No, I was never . . . Before I got married I used to sleep a lot. Once I stayed up through one whole night because I had a lot of work to do and then I slept for twenty-four hours.

Dr Detinis: Before the problem with your spine, in which position did you sleep?

Patient: In the foetal position.

Dr Detinis: How exactly?

Patient: Face down, one leg stretched out and the other . . .

Dr Detinis: Do you always sleep face down?

Patient: Yes, I love to sleep like that, I also sleep on my side.

Dr Detinis: Both positions?

Patient: Yes, but I usually prefer to sleep face down.

Dr Detinis: Do you have a recurring dream?

Patient: No, no, I never dream.

Dr Detinis: You never have done?

Patient: I never dream. Actually, I did have a dream recently, perhaps three days ago.

Dr Detinis: An unusual question: Have you ever felt telepathic or had any similar experiences?

Patient: Yes, like thinking of a person and then getting a call from them, or . . .

Dr Detinis: Anything more significant?

Patient: Yes, it was telepathy or something like that when I . . . three or four days before the first operation I woke up and . . . I decided not to tell my husband but I did tell him in the end. I dreamt of the neuro-surgeon who was going to operate on me and he said: 'Right, here are two swimming pools' – I was on a motorbike – and he said, 'Here are two swimming pools, if you get into the first one then you're on your own, but if you get into the other then I'll be there.' My husband said 'Don't let them operate on you.' I don't know if it was a premonition or what . . . I don't know.

Dr Detinis: Do you mind if my colleagues ask you a few questions?
Patient: Of course not, please do!

QUESTIONS FROM THE FLOOR

Question: Could you please tell us something about your pregnancies?
Patient: My pregnancies . . . the first one was straightforward, there weren't any complications. I was working right up to the last minute. We had just moved into our new flat and I wanted to get everything sorted out, and I didn't have any problems of any kind. During the second one, though, I was always losing blood. I had . . . I felt so weak all the time. I had to rest a lot because when I stood up I lost blood. The placenta was very low – they thought it might be *placenta praevia* but in the end it wasn't.

Question: Apart from the problems with your spine, what would you like to be cured of?
Patient: It's not just my spine, my whole body is in this awful state! . . . My whole body is out of order, there's my weight problem, my neurological problem, my gynaecological problem . . . I don't know where to begin, as I'm always saying to my friends.

Question: What sort of people do you dislike?
Patient: People who are deceitful or who don't listen to me when I talk to them.

Question: What makes you cry?
Patient: Well, as you may have heard when I told the doctor, it upsets me to talk about my brother and my daughters. Having a mother who's not well is the worst thing in the world. It's not my suffering so much as theirs, and I don't want them to suffer on my behalf.

Question: How do you feel right now?
Patient: I wish you could know what I was going through – it's hell! I'm covered in sweat, I itch and burn all over, because the itching makes my legs and back and my head and whole body burn . . . The first neurologist who treated me, the famous one, said that the perspiration along my spine was caused by pruritus of the femoral skin. The traumatologist noticed it, and then the neurologist confirmed it.

149

Dr Detinis: What was their diagnosis of the fibromas?

Patient: The uterus was enlarged, the fibromas are ball-shaped miomas inside at the back, and I've got one on the left which is bigger than the one on the right. The cyst is on the left ('Generalities, side, left' (1401/I).)

Question: What size is the cyst?

Patient: The miomas were about three centimetres in diameter when they did the last scan – I think that was in December.

COMMENTARY

At the beginning of the consultation the patient launched into a seemingly interminable account of her problems, which appeared to contain little of note. In fact this gives us our first symptom, 'Loquacity' (63/I). Her narrative was peppered with anecdotes and digressions, such as conversations she had with her doctors, and she demonstrated a prodigious memory. (These characteristics belong to a symptom I have frequently observed in patients who are of the constitutional type that I believe this woman to be, and to which I will return later on.) A second symptom was the curious tendency to repeat certain words and phrases – a symptom which appears in the *Synthetic Repertory*: 'Speech, repeats same thing' (column 943).

She showed herself to be extremely knowledgeable about her symptoms and diagnoses, although not in the manner of a Lycopodium patient, who tries to impress you with his erudition. There was no trace of pomposity or pedantry about her. This woman has a deep understanding of her problem and a strong command of all the technical terms relating to her illness.

The patient did not give us many mental or general symptoms. She appears to have concealed important aspects of her personality in her desire to be the perfect mother. Nevertheless, some of the typical characteristics of the remedy emerge; coquetry, for example. She said that her daughter's friends thought her young enough to be the sister, and not the mother, of the girl. Elsewhere the patient recalled that another friend had said, 'Your Mummy's so pretty'. Further evidence for this symptom is her fondness of jewelry and a sun-tan.

This woman has no doubts or worries, she is sure of herself to the point of being overconfident. The symptom in Kent's *Repertory* is 'Positiveness' (69/II). Many patients claim to be very self-confident, although one can see that they are basically insecure. But that is clearly not so in this case. Imagine the blow this woman must have suffered when, having been so hard-working and active, she was forced to retire three years ago because of her disability. Besides being a housewife, she held two teaching posts. The symptom that covers this is 'Industrious' (56/I). One final symptom is the desire for vengeance. Many patients who undergo spinal operations do not recover completely, but they do not retain, especially after so long a time, such a marked degree of malice. The patient said, 'If I get hold of that surgeon, I'll kill him!' and 'I'll make him pay for it!'.

As far as general symptoms are concerned, the only one that really stands out is the total absence of perspiration (we should ignore the perspiration she currently experiences, which is caused by her pathological condition.) This is 'Skin, inactivity' (1326/II). There is also a predominance of the left side, with a fibroma and an ovarian cyst on this side.

REPERTORISATION

'Positiveness' (69/II)
'Industrious' (56/I)
'Loquacity' (63/I)
'Malicious' (63/II)
'Skin, inactivity' (1326/II)

Prescription: Lachesis 1M.

Although Lachesis does not appear under 'Coquettish' in the *Synthetic Repertory*, in my personal experience it is one of the most frequently indicated remedies for the symptom. Lachesis women are very fond of necklaces, big jangly rings, brightly-coloured clothes, and they often dye their hair. They tend to conceal their age, wanting to seem younger than they really are. For several years I carried out clinical investigations as to which remedies have the greatest fear of growing old. Lachesis came first, with Lycopodium and Sepia in second place.

Another curious characteristic frequently observed in Lachesis women is their propensity to believe that young and handsome men find them sexually attractive. I remember the case of one woman in her seventies who told me that after she was widowed she was relentlessly pursued by the janitor in her block of flats, thirty years her junior, and also by the chemist, who used to 'say things to her'. She said that she had to put him in his place because he was in danger of overstepping the bounds of propriety.

I have also observed that Lachesis is fond of cats, superstitious (which I suggest should be added to the *Repertory*), and that Lachesis mothers are very possessive of their children.

FOLLOW-UP

(Two months after the first prescription)

Patient: After taking the remedy I had some symptoms that really frightened me. My legs went all weak and they were terribly, terribly itchy – the burning sensation I had before turned into an itch. For about two hours I felt like I had caught flu and my nose was very runny. I had bouts of nausea and I lost the strength in my legs. The pain in my spine and my waist got much worse. That all lasted for about a week and then I started to feel better. The terrible burning sensation on waking that I told you about didn't come back. I used to take a tranquilliser to relieve the itching and the sweating and for a whole month I didn't need to take it. My legs felt much stronger and the crawling sensation hasn't come back. I get the impression that the remedy worked – I began to be able to walk four or five blocks in town. My mobility improved by 40 per cent. My mood changed completely because I was feeling so much better. So I asked my husband and kids to take me out for a coffee and they were amazed and said, 'Mum, what did they give you?' I was able to walk with much more confidence, and I started having lots of dreams, which I never did before. What I notice now is how little muscle tone I have in my legs.

Case III: Jorge G., aged 32, married, one daughter aged five

Dr Detinis: Tell me what brings you here.

Patient: My problem goes back twelve years – I've got high cholesterol and lipid levels. My feet and hands swell up, I need a lot of sleep, and still feel very tired all the time. I get indigestion, and I smoke a lot.

Dr Detinis: How much do you smoke?

Patient: A packet, maybe a packet and a half a day, which is a lot considering that I had problems with my lungs – asthma – when I was a child. My left arm and part of my left leg seem to be sort of asleep. I also get tachycardia from time to time. I don't know if you're interested in the cholesterol figures . . .

Dr Detinis: Yes, I was just going to ask you about that.

Patient: I've brought the analysis.

Dr Detinis: Are you on medication?

Patient: I was taking medication which . . . You see, I've been treated by several doctors over the years so I've taken quite a lot of different medicines, but the last one was Lurselle. I've noticed that if I stop smoking the cholesterol level seems to come down a bit.

Dr Detinis: But at the moment you're not taking any medicines?

Patient: No, I'm not taking any, and maybe that's why my cholesterol level has gone up again. To be honest, I have to walk twenty-five blocks in a day's work and I just don't have the time. Well, it's not that I don't have the time, it's just that there's always something else to do, and so . . . I come home feeling shattered, and . . . Apart from that I was also put on a diet, but now this . . . I'm very greedy, I love food.

Dr Detinis: What kind of food?

Patient: Mainly sweet things ('Desires sweets' (486/II)).

Dr Detinis: Are you very fond of sweet things?

Patient: Yes, very, although I take saccharine in my coffee.

Dr Detinis: Which illnesses have you had apart from asthma?

Patient: Well, ones like chickenpox . . . in fact all of them except for scarlet fever, whooping cough and hepatitis.

Dr Detinis: Have you had any problems with your skin?

Patient: No, I've got a wart, and I also used to have a mole on my back. My wife works at the hospital so I went along to have it checked out. They removed it but they said it wasn't anything important, but there's a sort of tugging feeling here in my back. Apart from that I've

... my back is all tense, because I get up ... My wife says, 'If you sleep ... ' Well I do, but I always wake up feeling worse than when I went to bed.

Dr Detinis: Tell me what happens when you get up in the morning.
Patient: It takes a tremendous effort to get out of bed, and I ache all over, my back aches, and I try to stretch out and, well, you can hear my bones creaking now.

Dr Detinis: You said that you always feel tired. Do you find that it takes you a while to wake up in the morning, and you feel as though you were still half asleep?
Patient: Yes, the alarm clock rings and just goes on ringing ... ('Sleep, waking difficult' (1255/II)).

Dr Detinis: And then you sit up in bed and you still feel half asleep?
Patient: Yes – I don't really wake up until I've had a shower.

Dr Detinis: How long do you sleep?
Patient: Eight hours. I sleep but I don't feel refreshed ('Sleep, unrefreshing' (1254/II)).

Dr Detinis: In which position do you sleep?
Patient: On my right-hand side, with my arm under the pillow and my head on top.

Dr Detinis: Do you ever sleep on your left-hand side?
Patient: No, because I feel like I'm suffocating when I do that 'Respiration, difficult, lying on the left side' (770/I).

Dr Detinis: You find it hard to breathe?
Patient: Exactly. I had a series of injections for this bronchial problem I had when I was a child – I think they helped a bit, but they didn't cure it. I think if I stopped smoking I would be alright.

Dr Detinis: Do you have a recurring dream?
Patient: Do you mean nightmares?

Dr Detinis: Nightmares or any other dream that you have on different occasions.
Patient: No.

Dr Detinis: What about when you were a child?
Patient: Yes, there was something, though it was very strange. I dreamt I was by a jetty, in a boat that was hanging above the sea – that's why I said it was strange – and I was there inside the boat.

Dr Detinis: What do you mean 'a boat that was hanging above the sea?'

Patient: I was swinging inside this boat, without touching the water. I had that dream several times when I was a boy.

Dr Detinis: What line of work are you in?

Patient: I'm a representative for a company that makes windows and doors.

Dr Detinis: And how are things going?

Patient: Well, the construction industry is going through a bad patch, but I get by, you know.

Dr Detinis: How long have you been doing that?

Patient: One year. A year ago I was just about to emigrate. I've got a brother who's in Italy – he's my best friend, really – and well, what with the way things were a year ago, he invited me over to try my luck in Italy. I had already booked my passage, got an Italian visa.

Dr Detinis: How many brothers and sisters have you got?

Patient: Just the one brother, the one in Italy.

Dr Detinis: Is he older than you?

Patient: No, three years younger, he's twenty-nine.

Dr Detinis: And what about your family?

Patient: There's my wife and one daughter.

Dr Detinis: And how do you get on with them and with your parents?

Patient: I get on extremely well with my wife and daughter, though we sometimes have arguments like all married people do. With my parents . . . very well with my mother, not so well with my father, especially as I work in the same company as him.

Dr Detinis: Why don't you get on so well with your father, if I might ask?

Patient: Well, we just don't agree about anything.

Dr Detinis: Why, what's your father like? Tell me about him.

Patient: Well, he's rather conservative, but I admire him. I think I have a lot to learn from him, but we just don't agree – there's quite a character clash.

Dr Detinis: How can you admire him if you don't agree on anything?

Patient: At work, at the factory, we get on better, but at home we can't talk about anything because we are diametrically opposed . . .

Dr Detinis: Do you argue?

Patient: Yes, we argue; we argue but we never shout . . . well, hardly ever, not like in other families. I think I was rather rebellious when I was a boy and I used to get smacked quite a lot.

Dr Detinis: Did you deserve it?
Patient: I suppose so.

Dr Detinis: Why did you say that you were rebellious as a boy?
Patient: I was terrible, by all accounts; I got up to all sorts of awful things . . . Like hitting my brother, that was one of the things I often got punished for.

Dr Detinis: Why did you hit your brother?
Patient: I don't know, probably because he had a toy or something that I wanted at the time.

Dr Detinis: Were you a rather aggressive boy? Were you violent?
Patient: Yes, yes, all the time.

Dr Detinis: Towards your brother or towards children in general?
Patient: Mostly towards my brother, but I used to fight other children too.

Dr Detinis: When you were at primary school, did you work hard, what was your behaviour like?
Patient: I was good, although I was quite shy away from home.

Dr Detinis: How long did you stay at school?
Patient: I finished secondary school and then I started to study systems analysis, but I dropped out. That was another of the reasons why my father . . . Once he actually told me that I was a failure because I had dropped out ('Confidence, want of self') (13/II)).

Dr Detinis: Why did you drop out?
Patient: Because I wasn't enjoying it.

Dr Detinis: Was it your father who persuaded you to go into higher education?
Patient: Well, I think that every father wants his children to get an education. It's the only thing they can give them apart from love . . .

Dr Detinis: But after secondary school you can choose.
Patient: I could choose which subject but . . .

Dr Detinis: Choose to work or to study, and which subject you want to study.
Patient: Yes, you're right. I think I'd also try to get my daughter to go to college.

Dr Detinis: And why do your father's words stay in your mind – because it's some time since he said them?
Patient: Yes, but I can even remember the time and the place.

Dr Detinis: Why did it make such an impression on you?

Case III: Jorge G., aged 32, married, one daughter aged five

Patient: It must be because I don't want to be a failure ('Confidence, want of self').

Dr Detinis: Is that what you feel like?

Patient: Perhaps I did feel like that, perhaps I don't really like anything about myself. For example, my wife was head of public relations at Austral and it was really nice to see how happy she was when she came back from work . . . and I didn't have . . . But if you asked me now whether I'm happy with what I'm doing then I would say yes.

Dr Detinis: Are you content with what you're doing?

Patient: At the moment, yes.

Dr Detinis: What other memories do you have of your childhood, what were you like as a child? What feelings did you have towards your father, your mother, your brother . . . ?

Patient: I didn't have very good feelings towards my father, perhaps because he had a very important job at Esso in Campana and was away from home a lot. We knew he was our father but . . . we saw more of our mother. I remember something that my mother said, which was that I tried to get closer to him, but that he rejected me.

Dr Detinis: He rejected you?

Patient: That's what it felt like.

Dr Detinis: Why?

Patient: I don't know.

Dr Detinis: When did this happen?

Patient: Well, things began to improve when I got married and my wife came to live with us – I don't know what she had to do with it – but I noticed that things began to improve from then on.

Dr Detinis: Do you mean to say that you felt like this until your wife came to live with you?

Patient: Yes.

Dr Detinis: And it affected you?

Patient: Yes, of course!

Dr Detinis: Why ever did it happen?

Patient: I don't know, I suppose it was because I used to get smacked a lot. Then when I was a bit older I used to try to ask his advice about things and well, he didn't pay attention to me . . . Mostly I used to ask my mother about things.

Dr Detinis: Your father wasn't very interested in you?

Patient: No.

Dr Detinis: How did your father get on with your brother?

Patient: There weren't really any problems. Well, I suppose he was the favourite, but he wasn't as rebellious as me, he was quieter.

Dr Detinis: Apart from hitting your brother, in what other ways were you rebellious?

Patient: I don't know, I really don't know.

Dr Detinis: What are you like now?

Patient: I think that I'm fairly cheerful despite everything, but whenever I feel down I need a lot of support from my wife ('Confidence, want of self').

Dr Detinis: What do you mean by 'feeling down'?

Patient: It's how I feel when something has gone wrong.

Dr Detinis: You get depressed?

Patient: Yes, exactly.

Dr Detinis: And when you feel like that, what do you do? Do you cry, do you want to be by yourself?

Patient: No, I try to talk things over with my wife, or I sit down in an armchair at home, put the headphones on and listen to some classical music.

Dr Detinis: What happens when you listen to classical music?

Patient: Well, it's something which ... Sometimes I get more depressed and other times I lose myself and escape ... Another thing I have is that my memory is not very good.

Dr Detinis: Why did you link music with memory?

Patient: I don't know, it just came into my head.

Dr Detinis: How do you feel about music?

Patient: I don't know – I mainly like music by Bach and Vivaldi, because it cheers me up when I'm depressed, although sometimes it gets me down even more, but at least I spend an hour or so with my mind on something else.

Dr Detinis: And when you're not depressed, what effect does music have on you?

Patient: A pleasant one.

Dr Detinis: You like it, it makes you happy. Do you ever cry when you listen to music?

Patient: No, I don't, I'm not used to crying.

Dr Detinis: You don't ever cry?

Patient: No, I don't, but ... there are times when I really would like to in order to get some relief.

Dr Detinis: Do you often listen to music? Is it one of your hobbies?

Patient: No, my hobby at the moment is a personal computer that I bought.

Dr Detinis: What else can you say about your character?

Patient: I don't know.

Dr Detinis: Anything you can think of . . . ?

Patient: I don't know. I like to help my friends, something like that, I don't know. I always try to be . . . at those times, such as . . . unfortunately, I mean fortunately, we have lots of friends. Our weekends are always a write-off, we never manage to do all the things we arranged to do. We try to see people, go out with them, share their problems . . . other people's problems, see if we can help . . .

Dr Detinis: What would your wife say you were like?

Patient: You'd have to ask her that.

Dr Detinis: There's a point to the question – I want you to try and look at yourself objectively for a moment.

Patient: My wife says . . . I'm, well, basically . . . very fussy about tidiness and hygiene ('Conscientious about trifles' (16/I)). I've often said that even if I were blind I would know the exact whereabouts of everything in my room. What else would she say? I don't know, I think that ultimately I try to be a good husband. I've got my faults, mind you.

Dr Detinis: What are your faults?

Patient: Well actually . . . I'm laughing because I'm a bit nervous, all this is making me feel nervous.

Dr Detinis: The idea is to help you.

Patient: Of course, mind you I never enjoyed acting or being on a stage when I was at school.

Dr Detinis: Why, what did you feel?

Patient: Shy . . . what were we talking about? I'm sorry I was . . .

Dr Detinis: About your faults.

Patient: Oh, my faults? I don't know, perhaps I am a bit of an . . . egoist I don't know, I couldn't say whether I really was or not, I think I probably am a bit, deep down. But . . . how should I know! ('Selfishness' (78/I)).

Dr Detinis: What makes you think that?

Patient: Because I once got a terrible shock when they took me to the doctor when I had an asthma attack, and the doctor told me that if I carried on smoking . . .

Dr Detinis: Why do you think you could be an egoist?

Patient: I don't know, perhaps because I want to live as much as possible and forget about everyone else. I don't know, because that contradicts what I said before about sharing other people's problems and trying to help them. I really don't know. I suppose I am a bit of an egoist. ('Selfishness').

Dr Detinis: You said that you were shy. How did you feel when you had to take exams?

Patient: Terribly insecure ('Confidence, want of self').

Dr Detinis: Did you have any symptoms just before exams?

Patient: Not that I remember. Nerves, but that's quite normal isn't it?

Dr Detinis: When you have an emotion, do you feel it in any particular part of your body?

Patient: What kind of an emotion?

Dr Detinis: A fright, a fit of temper, something like that.

Patient: I think it affects my heartbeat.

Dr Detinis: These tachycardias you mentioned?

Patient: Yes, or my ears burn.

Dr Detinis: Just your ears?

Patient: Perhaps my face goes red too, but I feel it most in my ears.

Dr Detinis: From what kind of emotion?

Patient: Shyness ('Timidity, bashful' (89/I)).

Dr Detinis: Are you scared of anything?

Patient: Yes, of the dark and heights.

Dr Detinis: What happens to you in the dark?

Patient: I don't know, I think that . . . I don't know. I'm scared of the dark, and also . . . of thunder. That's very childish, isn't it?

Dr Detinis: Not really, we all have certain fears.

Patient: Well, for example, most people are scared of death but I find I'm more scared of the idea of being put in a coffin.

Dr Detinis: Why?

Patient: Because you're shut away in the darkness. I'm not claustrophobic because I don't mind using a lift, as long as there's light there's no problem. I'm scared of the dark . . . or rather, I'm scared that I'll see things in the dark, strange things, monsters like I used to see when I was a child.

Case III: Jorge G., aged 32, married, one daughter aged five

Dr Detinis: Did you see things like that?

Patient: I saw them a few times and there was a television programme that I couldn't put out of my mind . . .

Dr Detinis: But you didn't imagine them?

Patient: No, I suppose after I'd seen a film, in the dark . . .

Dr Detinis: What sort of things did you see?

Patient: That kind of thing.

Dr Detinis: Something you had already seen?

Patient: Yes, I've got a bad memory for facts, but a very good visual memory.

Dr Detinis: And did you only see faces, or bodies too?

Patient: Mainly faces, horrible faces. For example, the other day I saw a magazine, I don't know which one because it wasn't mine . . . it didn't scare me, but there was a photograph of some children that . . . It shook me. I put it back at once ('Delusions, faces, sees hideous' (25/I)). ('Horrible things, sad stories, affect her profoundly' (52/I)).

Dr Detinis: Do you sleep with a light on?

Patient: No.

Dr Detinis: Do you feel scared above a certain height?

Patient: Yes. We own a mill out in the countryside, a ruined old mill. Once I climbed up to the top and then I had to step down in order to get down on to this platform. I held on and came down, then I felt dizzy and . . . because that's another thing . . . I get strange feelings, blackouts . . . it's as though something lifted me up and put me down, it's a strange feeling.

Dr Detinis: In those circumstances?

Patient: Not only then, when I'm feeling calm too.

Dr Detinis: Do you have any other fears?

Patient: I faint whenever I see blood; I often faint when I have to give a blood sample ('Horrible things').

Dr Detinis: Any other fears – dogs, for instance?

Patient: Well, I have quite a healthy respect for dogs, but I'm not scared of them. What I'm scared of is that the dog might bite me and then I'd see blood.

Dr Detinis: So it would be more true to say that you're impressionable because if I showed you a little puppy . . .

Patient: Yes, that's right. If I were to give my daughter a little dog I wouldn't be scared, not of a dog like that.

Dr Detinis: Are you scared of thieves, of being alone?

Patient: Yes, but I've been robbed . . .

Dr Detinis: And before then?

Patient: No, because I thought I could fight them off.

Dr Detinis: How do you feel when you're alone in the house?

Patient: I don't like to be alone.

Dr Detinis: What do you feel?

Patient: I really don't like it, perhaps because I'm scared at night, although I used to have to travel at certain times and then I'd be alone, staying at a hotel . . . It's not a fear – I just don't like to be alone.

Dr Detinis: How loving are you?

Patient: With my wife, my mother and my daughter, the people who are closest to me, I'm very loving; I try to be, with my father, but there's something . . .

Dr Detinis: Are you very affectionate, do you kiss them . . . ?

Patient: Yes, yes, yes.

Dr Detinis: Are you on top of them all day long?

Patient: Yes.

Dr Detinis: So much so that they start to get annoyed?

Patient: No, I don't think it annoys them. I think that if my brother was here I would be like that with him too, hugging him . . .

Dr Detinis: In what circumstances do you feel jealous?

Patient: Never. I was very jealous before I was married, of my wife; but it was the loving kind of jealousy. Otherwise, no.

Dr Detinis: Are you vindictive?

Patient: Not that I'm aware of. If anyone laid a finger on my family . . . because for me my family consists of my wife, my daughter, my mother, my father, my brother and an aunt, my grandmother died recently. If anyone laid a finger on any of them, I wouldn't be responsible for my actions. I'm very impulsive.

Dr Detinis: How do you mean, impulsive?

Patient: I mean I'd let out all the pent-up anger that I felt.

Dr Detinis: How would you do that?

Patient: Just by talking, did you think I meant physically?

Dr Detinis: I was asking you, not telling you.

Patient: No, I don't think that I'd hit anyone, I wouldn't like to mess up my clothes! But I don't think I'd take it that far, I've already been in that situation.

Case III: Jorge G., aged 32, married, one daughter aged five

Dr Detinis: Who or what is emotionally most important to you?
Patient: My brother.

Dr Detinis: Why do you feel so strongly about your brother?
Patient: I don't really know; he's my best friend. Whenever I talk about my brother . . . Life can be so cruel . . . You see, we got on badly for such a long time and suddenly just as we began to get on well he went away.

Dr Detinis: Why did you get on badly?
Patient: I think it was because we were both kids and I was terrible. I used to fill whole exercise books with 'I must not fight, I must not answer back, I must not . . .'

Dr Detinis: Were you made to do that at home?
Patient: Yes, it was a punishment, that or not being allowed to watch television.

Dr Detinis: Is there anything else that is emotionally important to you?
Patient: Not that I can think of right now.

Dr Detinis: You said that you have a sweet tooth. What else do you like to eat?
Patient: Everything that makes me put on weight – I don't know if you've noticed! In the way of meat, I'm very fond of roasts, and I'd give my right arm for fried eggs or a potato omelette. I haven't had one for years!

Dr Detinis: You're very fond of eggs?
Patient: Fried eggs especially.

Dr Detinis: How many would you have?
Patient: I could eat any number, but . . . Just think, I haven't had any for nearly twelve years.

Dr Detinis: Do they disagree with you?
Patient: No, because of the cholesterol.

Dr Detinis: That's how long you've had a high cholesterol level?
Patient: Yes, because they first noticed it when I was doing my military service. I was bitten by an insect and I had a . . . I don't know how to put it so that you don't get me wrong. I did my military service in the San Martin Military District and, well, there are ways of getting round it . . . Someone told me what to do. I asked him to get me a dozen pastries (I love pastries too) and a corporal saw us – it was strictly forbidden. So I said it was all my fault and he was about to throw me into the lock-up. Well of course I didn't fancy not seeing my

family for a long time, and as I had this insect bite on my face, I managed to get a friend to have me admitted to the Military Hospital for two months . . . To cut a long story short they did all kinds of tests and discovered that I had a high cholesterol level.

Dr Detinis: What else do you like apart from sweet things?
Patient: Pasta, pumpkin in syrup, mayonnaise . . . You'd really have to ask me what I don't like.

Dr Detinis: Well, is there anything you don't like?
Patient: Yes, pork sausages, I can't even bear the smell of them.

Dr Detinis: Do you like spicy things?
Patient: I love them! You should have seen the fried eggs I used to make myself, all covered in sauces.

Dr Detinis: Sour things, vinegar, lemon?
Patient: I like vinegar, lemon not so much.

Dr Detinis: Animal fat?
Patient: I don't like it.

Dr Detinis: Milk, fish?
Patient: Milk yes, and I do eat fish but I don't like it because all the bones are so fiddly.

Dr Detinis: Cheese?
Patient: Yes, I eat it.

Dr Detinis: How hot do you like your food and drink?
Patient: I don't drink, just water.

Dr Detinis: Coffee, for example?
Patient: Lukewarm. I don't like it hot. I'm always in a hurry to eat, and if something's hot then I have to blow on it and wait . . .

Dr Detinis: What do you like least, the heat or the cold?
Patient: The heat, I think, but the only place I sweat is from the neck upwards, on my head ('Perspiration, only on the head' (222/I)).

Dr Detinis: When do you sweat on your head?
Patient: When it's very hot.

Dr Detinis: Does the weather affect you?
Patient: Generally I get a cold when there's a change in temperature and according to an allergy analysis I had done, I'm allergic to pollen, the fluff from plane trees and dust.

Dr Detinis: Does the sun affect you?
Patient: No.

Dr Detinis: Do you like being by the sea?
Patient: Yes, but I prefer the mountains.

Dr Detinis: When you're feeling 'down' and someone comes and consoles you, how do you feel?
Patient: Probably the only person I talk to is my wife, or if not her, then my brother, if he was there. I try to take their advice and act according to it even if it's not what I would want to hear.

QUESTIONS FROM THE FLOOR

Question: How do you react when someone contradicts you?
Patient: I always listen because I might be wrong, although I'm fairly stubborn and don't change my mind that easily, unless I really am wrong.

Question: How are you with money?
Patient: Ever since I got married I've kept accounts with graphs and everything for all my income and expenditures . . .

Question: Are you meticulous?
Patient: Very much so, where money is concerned.

Question: Why?
Patient: I just like it. I once worked out how much money I should have at the end of a six-month period and I wasn't even a penny out. I don't live badly, I could live better, but I think that the current economic situation is pretty bad, especially in the building trade, where there's a recession at the moment.

Question: At one point you said that 'even if I was blind I would know exactly where everything in my room was'. Why did you say 'blind' and not 'if I had my eyes shut', because that seems to tie in with your fear of darkness. Are you worried about your sight?
Patient: I think I'd rather have my cholesterol problem than lose my sight.

Question: Do you have any problems with your digestion?
Patient: Yes, I get indigestion. I feel bloated and sick.

Question: How do you feel about the future?
Patient: I don't think about the future, I keep my mind on the present because I don't think I'll live much longer ('Doubtful, recovery, of' (37/1)).

Question: Why do you say that?
Patient: Because I've been trying to bring my cholesterol level down for twelve years without any success and rather than get arteriosclerosis . . . Don't get me wrong, because I would never be able to commit suicide.
Question: What's your aim in life?
Patient: To live in the here and now as much as I can.

COMMENTARY

Jorge has many characteristic symptoms. Which ones should we repertorise? Right at the beginning we came across three symptoms relating to sleep: 'Sleep, unrefreshing' (1254/II); 'Sleep, waking difficult' (1255/II); and 'Respiration, difficult, lying on the left side' (770/I).

Staying with the general symptoms, the patient has that anxious and excessive desire for food and sweet things that is typical of the symptom 'Gluttony' in the *Synthetic Repertory* (column 564). 'Perspiration, only on the head' (222/I) is an obvious symptom, clearly expressed by the patient.

Turning now to the mental symptoms, Jorge has an egoistic personality, which is 'Selfishness' (78/I). At two points during his account he gave himself away: 'I like to help my friends . . . unfortunately, I mean fortunately, we have lots of friends . . . ', and 'We try to share other people's problems . . . see if we can help them'.

Later however he said, 'I don't know, perhaps I am a bit of an egoist . . . I want to live as much as possible and forget about everyone else . . . I don't know, because that contradicts what I said before about trying to help other people.' His egoism is apparent from these conflicting statements. He regards his friends as little more than strangers.

He keenly felt his father's rejection and his lack of attention. His father hit him for being rebellious; he also suffered when his father was away on business. He told us, 'I tried to get closer to him but he rejected me . . . he didn't pay attention to me.'

Emotionally he is close only to his brother, whom he misses, and to his wife. He finds support in his wife. This need for support, combined with the 'complete insecurity' which he said he felt before exams, and the phrase of his father's that stayed fixed in his mind, and which he quoted to us – 'You're a failure' – constitutes one of Jorge's central symptoms: 'Confidence, want of self' (13/II).

Case III: Jorge G., aged 32, married, one daughter aged five

Jorge's strongest symptom, however, is a fear of the dark, so much so that his fear of death is actually a fear of the darkness of the coffin (he explained that this feeling was not one of claustrophobia). As a child he used to see horrible faces in the dark after watching films. This most interesting symptom is 'Delusions, faces, sees hideous' (25/I).

He is an impressionable patient, as is evident from his account of his reaction at seeing these children's faces in the magazine, and his propensity to faint at the sight of blood, or when giving blood.

He has many fears: of darkness, heights, storms, and so on.

Despite claiming to be very affectionate, he does not seem to be a loving person.

He has the symptom 'Conscientious about trifles' (16/I); on being asked what his wife would say about him he replied, 'I'm very fussy about tidiness and hygiene.' You will also remember that when one of you asked him how he was with money, he said he was very meticulous and that all his married life he had kept accounts of his income and expenditures. Finally, one symptom which appeared at the end was 'Doubtful, recovery, of' (37/I), or alternatively, 'Despair, recovery' (36/I). He does not believe that he will live much longer, because of his high cholesterol level.

REPERTORISATION

These are the symptoms that we must repertorise:

'Fear, dark' (43/II)
'Horrible things, sad stories, affect her profoundly' (52/I)
'Confidence, want of self' (13/II)
'Conscientious about trifles' (16/I)
'Perspiration, only on the head' (222/I)
'Waking, difficult' (1255/II)

Prescription: Calcarea Carbonica 1M. This is the only remedy which covers all the symptoms.

Case IV: Mrs E., aged 49, married, no children

Dr Detinis: Please tell me what brings you here.

Patient: I've had arthritis for nearly five years now. Five years ago I started to get terrible pains in the hip, and they got worse and worse. I went to see the doctor and he sent me to have some X-rays taken and he put me on medication. I wore a medical corset for three years and the pains more or less went away, but they do tend to come and go. I've got problems with my knees, elbows, hands and especially with my fingers and neck. The X-rays showed that there's also something wrong with my cervix, and in the lumbar region, and in the coccyx. And about three weeks ago an X-ray showed that I'm starting to get arthritis in the other hip too. The doctor says it's all getting worse, despite the fact that he's seen me so many times and given me so much medicine.

At the moment they're giving me iontophoresis, which does help to soothe the pain a bit, particularly in my hip. But sometimes I don't even have the strength in my elbows and fingers to pick things up. Usually when I wake up my hand is swollen – always the left one. I sometimes have bad headaches. I've taken an awful lot of tranquillisers and they calm me down, but it never goes away . . . I've also had massages . . . So the last time the doctor saw me he said: 'Look, I know where you can get some treatment that will hold up the process, though it's already very advanced. Go along and let's see what they have to say.'

Dr Detinis: And is there anything else?

Patient: Yes, there is. I've had tests which show that my uric acid level has been a bit high and I've been taking medication to bring it down.

Dr Detinis: Can you remember what the figures were?

Patient: About seven.

Dr Detinis: What are you taking for it?

Patient: Allopurinol. I've nearly finished a bottle of one hundred pills.

Dr Detinis: Have you brought the analysis with you?

Patient: No, I didn't know – I could have brought the X-rays too.

Dr Detinis: I want you to stop taking the pills and to bring me the analysis next time you see me. It's not a good idea to take other medication when you're being treated homoeopathically, and in any case I hope to be able to bring the uric acid down to its normal level. What else is there? Do you have any other symptoms?

Case IV: Mrs E., aged 49, married, no children

Patient: Well, I'm in almost constant pain and sometimes I can't raise my arms. At work I can't lean forward or bend down. I can't even put my clothes on because I haven't got any strength in my arms. I'm the headmaster's secretary at two different schools and I spend all day long in the office. I'm at my desk almost all the time and sometimes when I've been sitting for an hour I can hardly get up again . . . that's when things are very bad, because usually it gets me in one place or another, my hip, or my elbows, or my neck.

Dr Detinis: In different places?

Patient: Yes, in different places.

Dr Detinis: In different places each time?

Patient: I used to say that it seemed to go from one place to another, because sometimes my neck hurts a great deal, and sometimes my elbows, or my fingers, all of this area from here, which some-times makes it difficult for me to pick up things ('Pain, wandering' (1389/II)).

Dr Detinis: Have you noticed if these pains ever get better or worse for any reason?

Patient: I think it's just getting worse and worse because . . .

Dr Detinis: I don't mean better in the sense of disappearing, but just of easing off a little.

Patient: It gets better in one place and appears in another.

Dr Detinis: Such things as the weather, for instance; does it have anything to do with the time of year, or with anything else?

Patient: I've noticed that when I'm nervous the pains get worse. The damp is very bad for me, and so is the cold. I never used to get pains in the summer, but this year I was in a very, very bad state.

Dr Detinis: When you say 'nervous', what exactly do you mean?

Patient: When I have to deal with an important situation at work, something which hasn't been done properly. Nothing terribly impor-tant, just things that I get worried or upset about . . . I tend to worry too much about things that don't get done or which I have to sort out because someone else didn't do them properly. That's when the pains get worse.

Dr Detinis: Do you mean you have to do other people's jobs for them?

Patient: Exactly!

Husband: She is very conscientious about fulfilling her responsibilities and the staff don't always do things properly or on time. She's not used to making mistakes because she's so meticulous, and if everything doesn't go according to plan she gets upset and feels tense.

Patient: Yes, I get tense. I've been going to a masseur for a while. It helps a lot because when I get very tense, my neck gets all knotted up – she actually pointed out where it was knotty in my neck and in this part of my back. The massages help a lot because they relax me. I should learn to relax a bit more and not get so tense.

Husband: This summer her pains were much worse because she was feeling emotionally very tense about a relative of hers who was dying. She was in a great deal of distress.

Patient: My feet and legs were very swollen.

Dr Detinis: Do tell me about your relative.

Patient: It was an aunt of mine who had had a stroke, an old lady who was almost a mother to me, and to whom I was very close. We were in Cordoba at the time. We couldn't stay with her and so we had to travel a long way each time we went to see her.

Dr Detinis: Where was she?

Patient: She was in Villa Maria. All the travelling aggravated the pain so much that in the end I just couldn't walk.

Dr Detinis: How else did this situation affect you, and why?

Patient: I was upset that I couldn't be with her all the time, I couldn't stay with her because it was impossible. It was that, and all the travelling, and the fact that I could see there was nothing to be done because she had had a stroke and each time we saw her she was . . .

Husband: At the beginning the weather was terribly hot, and this place is high up in the mountains. Within a week she was very dehydrated and she had an intestinal infection that didn't clear up for a long time. She was quite ill.

Dr Detinis: I want you to explain all this, because it might help us to understand you better. I will also ask you questions (addressing her husband), because you can help with things that might not occur to your wife. How did you feel in this situation?

Patient: I felt very tense, very ill, very upset. I couldn't help in any way. I could see that her condition was deteriorating each day and there was nothing to be done; she was eighty years old and dying. At one point I thought I'd lose my mind . . . I was terribly upset . . .

Dr Detinis: What exactly did you find distressing about this situation?

Patient: I couldn't do anything to help, apart from help financially, but not really . . . ('Anxiety, conscience, of (as if guilty of a crime)' (6/I)). The doctor said that nothing could be done to save her, that she was dying . . . We tried to do all we could for her, and of course we did, we did, I know we did all that is humanly possible, all that one could do for a loved one. And all this travelling . . . She died in March, while we were here in Buenos Aires. It was during term-time and we rushed over there to be with her but it was too late . . .

Dr Detinis: You weren't at her side?

Patient: Not when she died, but just after that . . .

Dr Detinis: On the deepest level, what were your feelings about the situation? You said that this lady was like a mother to you.

Patient: She brought me up from a very early age.

Dr Detinis: I would like you to tell us about that in a moment, but first I'd like to ask you about something that both you and your husband mentioned. You said that most of all you were upset because you couldn't do anything to help her. Was there an underlying feeling in you that you can tell me about?

Patient: No, no, I meant that we could see she was dying and we made sure she received medical attention, we took her to hospital, and then when they discharged her we put her in a nursing home, paid for everything, stayed by her side . . . It was just the grief of knowing that there was simply nothing else that could be done for her.

Dr Detinis: But why did you question this, why do you doubt it, that's what I don't understand.

Patient: I didn't question it, I just meant that one sometimes feels helpless because one sees that one can't help however much one tries, however much . . .

Dr Detinis: But did you at any time feel that you didn't do everything you could have done?

Patient: No, no, no. It was just the grief of losing a loved one that . . .

Dr Detinis: Tell me about yourself, your childhood, whether you have brothers and sisters. Tell me about your father and mother, about this aunt who was like a mother to you.

Patient: She was my mother's eldest sister. My parents separated when I was very young. She was my godmother and took me into her care. She didn't have any children and she treated me like a daughter for many years. Later, circumstances parted us for quite a long time and I was only able to see her on rare occasions. I married nearly five years ago, and then I began to see more of her, my husband always came with me. We tried to be with her as often as we could, and she was always overjoyed to see us.

Husband: I should like to add something which is quite important.

171

When this lady took my wife into her care, she was quite well off. She was married to a businessman and so her circumstances were quite different to those she had known as a child in Villa Maria, where her parents had been farmers ... But one summer when they were in Necochea together on holiday, the husband suddenly died of a heart attack. I believe that this had a profound effect on my wife – it left her feeling helpless and alone. So as I see it, the sorrow that she felt over her aunt was a natural reaction, a deeply-felt fear of the future and what it holds. So now whenever she has to deal with some problem or situation she gets tense and nervous. The death of her aunt is a prime example, but it's not the only one. For instance, something recently happened at school which brought on a nervous crisis and then she had to take sick-leave.

Dr Detinis: May I just interrupt you? What you have just told me is extremely valuable, but it's vital that your wife tells us these things in her own words.

Husband: Something upset her greatly ...

Patient: There was some trouble at the school, I had to make a formal report about the whole problem. It aggravated my condition, having to say lots of things that made me feel very bad, very tense and upset ... I was doing my duty, which of course one must, but I'm always afraid to. Sometimes I worry that something might happen to me, or he might go out and then if he doesn't come home on time I worry that something might have happened to him ... There's always this feeling of anxiety, of helplessness, fear that something might happen to me or to him ... ('Fear, happen, something will' (45/II)).

Dr Detinis: Do you fear that something might happen to you?

Patient: It's him I usually worry about. When he leaves the house I'll tell him over and over again to take care of himself, and if he's late I worry that something has happened to him. It's a natural response, I'm always worrying about what will happen ...

Dr Detinis: Can you be more precise?

Patient: I worry that something could happen to us, to him, or to me.

Dr Detinis: What kind of thing?

Patient: Something ... I don't know! We haven't been married long and I always have this fear that something will happen to him or to me, and he'll be left all alone ... I often worry about it.

Dr Detinis: With regard to what, an accident, your health?

Patient: Well, for instance there are lots of things I should do round the house which I can't do. Unfortunately I have to depend on the lady who comes and does the housework for me. I can't clean the floors or do the washing. My husband is very supportive but I feel so anxious and always worry that one of these days I won't be any more use to him. One of the first doctors to treat me told me that if I hadn't come to see him then I could have ended up in a wheelchair. It gave me quite a shock, as you can imagine. That was when I had to wear the corset, but after two years they took it off because I couldn't stand it any more.

Dr Detinis: Do continue in this way, you're doing very well. You see, although your husband could tell us all this, the most important thing is what you feel, not what someone else thinks you feel. You might have a different opinion to the one your husband has of you. Forget the words he used, which were probably originally yours anyway. I want you to go on telling us about your childhood. You mentioned the fact that your parents separated when you were young. How old were you then?

Patient: I think my parents separated . . . I don't actually remember when, it was my aunt who told me. I think I was about eighteen months. My mother and father separated and she had custody.

Dr Detinis: Didn't you go to your aunt?

Patient: They separated and my aunt saw that we were alone and as she was my godmother she took me into her home. My sister stayed with my mother and I went to my aunt.

Dr Detinis: Is your sister older or younger than you?

Patient: She's fifty-three, four years older than me. We separated and for a long time we never saw each other again.

Dr Detinis: Who do you mean?

Patient: My mother and my sister.

Dr Detinis: How old were you then?

Patient: I didn't see either my mother or my sister from the age of about eighteen months until I was fourteen, while I lived with my aunt. Then . . .

Dr Detinis: Why didn't you see your mother for such a long time?

Patient: The sisters – my mother and my aunt that is – broke off relations. I don't know why, when my mother and father had just separated . . . I think that my aunt came and saw us, we were just two little girls, and she took me to live with her and never brought me back to my mother's house, and I never went back myself because, well, I was just a little girl. That's how it was. I entered a convent at the age of fourteen.

Dr Detinis: When did see your mother again?
Patient: Well, I saw my mother the day I took the veil. The day I took the veil my mother . . . It was like this: while I was a novice I was in contact only with my aunt. One day I had to apply for some document or other and I wrote to the Register Office to ask for my birth certificate, but for some unknown reason they sent it to my sister instead. So I wrote to my aunt, with whom I was in touch, and she told me, 'Your mother is living in Villa Maria with your sister'. So I found their address and I wrote to my mother and told her that I was in a convent and that I was going to take the vows in December, and that I should like to see her. But she didn't reply and I didn't know whether they were coming or not. After the ceremony, everyone is supposed to greet their family; I didn't know if anyone other than my aunt would be there . . . But I looked round the convent and suddenly I heard my mother calling me and then there she was with me again . . . I was fourteen years old. And we all started to see each other again; they always came to visit me . . . and on the few occasions when I was allowed to leave the convent, I went to see them. Well, I got quite close to my mother and to my sister too; she married and came here to Buenos Aires and has children. I left the convent in 1974.

Dr Detinis: Why did you become a nun?
Patient: Why? I don't really know why . . . I think that at that time I really thought it was my vocation. I managed to do many things as a nun, with much enthusiasm and much love, because when I do something, I do it with all my heart – that's why I worry and suffer so much. I studied teacher training in Spanish language and literature and completely dedicated myself to it. I was a form teacher, a nursery school teacher and I taught a lot of different subjects before I completed the training and had to specialise. I rose to be principal of a secondary school, and headmistress of a primary school . . . a bit of everything.

But I soon realised that many things were not actually as I would have wished them to be, and finally it got to a point where I was not living the life I wanted to. There were many things I had to do, being in a position of authority, many things which I could not reconcile with my own nature. When one is in a position of authority one sometimes has to deal with the staff, you have to try to see every point of view. For example, I have the satisfaction of meeting women who are teachers now, whom I knew when they were doing their teacher training with me. I have always got on very well with the people under me – with my colleagues, that is – even though I was in a position of authority. Yet I couldn't see everything clearly at the time, and there was much injustice at work that I could not put up with ('Indignation' (55/II)).

I was always scared of leaving the convent. Life as a nun involves a whole process of training, though with hindsight I can see that things aren't quite as we were led to believe. The Christian life, the life of people who believe in God and who care for other people, is more . . . it isn't as full of petty rules and regulations; the injustice and lack of charity in the convent was intolerable ('Indignation'). There was much injustice and a great deal of misunderstanding, and I realised I couldn't go on like that. And now that I have a home, a husband and a house to look after, I can see that the life of the layman is also full of sacrifices and effort and full of love, and that there are very virtuous people among the laity too. I began to see this, and I began to understand it, and I said, 'Right, whether I leave the convent or not, I will be truer to myself and a better person, and my life will be more real, because I don't like what I'm doing here.'

I was always afraid of leaving, and always tried to appease this fear by looking for something to keep me occupied in my job as head-teacher. As a teacher, I was always looking for something to organise, something to do. I think I had to do this to silence the small voice that was telling me, 'You can't stay here', because I didn't feel at ease with myself; but I was scared to face up to life. And I remember that in the first few months after I left I thought that everyone was looking at me all the time, that everyone knew I had been a nun, and I suffered a great deal. But in fact those who knew me, who welcomed me, those who had been with me when I was a nun and who now saw me as one of the laity and later as a married woman, were very fond of me and remembered me with much love after I had left the convent.

I had to overcome a very great fear, so when an opportunity arose – that's not to say I'm an opportunist, I think that God gave me the chance to leave – I seized it. There was a serious crisis in the Sister-hood to which I belonged, and it was dissolved. So I said, 'Right, this is my chance' because then I had the strength to say, 'I'm leaving' and so I did. It was very difficult for me because I had to drop a lot of long-term plans. So much so that, although I have now got over it, until recently I often used to dream that I was still a nun and that I was walking and walking without any shoes and with an empty bag . . . I dreamt that many times; I think it's a way of freeing oneself from all of that. Now I don't have that dream so often, but at first . . . It was a very great struggle to leave; because of course, it's much easier to stay and to lead a comfortable life in the convent, and just accept a whole lot of things, and have everything taken care of, because everything is there for you, than to have to face up to life and to say, 'I'm leaving' and then to have to find work.

I spent months and months looking for work, knocking on one door after another, but despite the fact that I was qualified I couldn't find any because no one knew me, and I had no relevant seniority. I had only taught in private schools and that didn't count when it came to state schools. It was very hard! My husband helped me a great deal, I owe him everything I have now. Many good things have happened, probably this state of anxiety, of fear and helplessness . . . I was afraid to leave because I was afraid of life, what was I to do alone in life? Then it was a great struggle to get married, it was terribly hard, not because of my husband . . . Because when I left I had to find some-where to stay, I had nowhere to go, I had no . . . I didn't want to stay at a boarding house. I was really alone.

I had been separated for so long from my sister that I didn't have the same sort of relationship with her as two sisters who have grown up together would have done. I regret not having had a normal and natural relationship with my sister, as I've often said to my husband. I love her very much and we see each other, we visit each other, but there isn't much . . . I think that was why. When I left, I could have said, 'I'll go and stay with my sister', but my life in the convent had separated us, had drawn us apart. I was a nun for almost twenty years, so you can imagine I was going through a whole . . . and when I left I had nowhere to go. I was offered a room in a house with two spinster sisters and their maid. One of these sisters worked in the school where I was headteacher, and she saw my position and said, 'Come and stay with us until you find something'. I stayed with them until I started to look for work, two very pleasant years. Then I realised that I had to sort something out because I couldn't spend the rest of my life there. And I think that secretly I had wanted to have a home and a companion in life. As a nun – I realise this now that I'm older – I was friends with all the girls, I used to enjoy teaching all the groups of girls . . . and they used to ask me, 'Don't you want to get married and have a family?' And I would tell them, 'No, I don't, I said no to all that when I became a nun.' But I realise that now that I am married and have a home (and although we don't have any children we are very happy), I now realise that perhaps that's what I really needed all along . . . I should have married instead of entering the convent.

Dr Detinis: So why did you enter the convent?
Patient: Well, because that's how things turned out. When my aunt lost her husband, she entered a convent for widows and put me in a school, a boarding school. I was just a little girl. And well, I wondered where I would go when I left school . . . my aunt had . . . she was the only person I had, I hadn't seen my mother, hadn't had any contact with her; the only person in my life was my aunt. My aunt entered a convent . . . I think it must have been all of those things, and I was just a girl at the time . . . So I decided to become a nun too . . . and everything followed on from there.

I found out from my aunt that my father was living in Ballesteros, and that he was very ill with a chronic myocarditis, that he had rheumatism and could hardly walk. He worked on the land, had his own smallholding . . . He had to work in all sorts of bad weather and it ruined his health. I found out where he was and wrote to him and of course he asked me to come and see him, but as novices we were not allowed to leave the convent, one had to wait until one had taken one's vows before being allowed to go out. He wrote to me, I wrote back to him, we began a correspondence. He was living with his elder sister who had two children; he could no longer write because his hands shook so much . . . And then his sister wrote to me and asked me to come and see them.

One day, after I had taken the vows, Mother Superior told me to accompany a Sister on a journey to Villa Maria, which is quite close to Ballesteros. Then she said, 'Look, you're not really supposed to go there, but since the two towns aren't far apart, take the bus with her, visit your father and then come straight back.' Well, so I went and saw my father for what was to all intents and purposes the first time because I hadn't seen him since he and my mother separated when I was just one year old. He was very ill, so much so that I said to his sister, 'Look, if his condition gets worse, please contact me at the convent because I think in those circumstances I would be allowed to come out and see him again.' That was on the 25th May. On the 8th June I received a telegram: 'Father seriously ill, come immediately.' Mother Superior handed me the telegram and said, 'Go quickly!' Someone went with me. When I arrived, Father had died. But at least I had had a chance to see him again.

Dr Detinis: And your adopted father?
Patient: My aunt's husband? He had died many years before in

Necochea, when I was four. My aunt was my godmother and her husband my godfather. He died on the beach in Necochea when I was four. I was in my twenties when my father died, and I had recently taken my vows.

Dr Detinis: I was struck by what your husband said about how much you were affected by the death of . . . who was it?

Patient: That was the same man, my uncle. He died on the beach and my aunt and I lived alone for many years. Then, when I was fourteen, she put me into a school, entered a convent for widows and I stayed at the school until I too entered a convent.

Dr Detinis: What did you feel when your aunt sent you to the boarding school?

Patient: I don't know what I felt at the time, I don't know, I don't have any particular memories of that. But once I was there I never wanted to leave again because I felt awful, terrible, I didn't think that I could manage alone . . . that's why I stayed on and on and tried to do as best I could as a nun, so that at least when I left I would have the satisfaction of knowing that I had worked with much enthusiasm, with much love and in a spirit of sacrifice.

Dr Detinis: What was the worst time of your life?

Patient: There were so many things! So many things happened while I was a nun. And when my aunt and I were left alone, she was quite well off financially. But she didn't have a job and there I was growing up alongside her and she was slowly running out of money. Even though I was only a child, I remember her going off to the bank each time until one day she came back and said, 'That's it, there's none left'. And I was terribly upset, I felt awful; perhaps that's where the feeling of helplessness came from ('Anxiety, future, about' (7/I)). Then she entered this sisterhood of widows and put me in this boarding school. When you enter a convent you have to bring a dowry and of course I didn't bring one and I was often reminded about it while I was there; I was always the one who hadn't brought a dowry, and when I left I didn't have a penny to my name.

Dr Detinis: Let's go back for a moment to the beginning of the conversation. You seem to have mixed feelings about the fact that your role, insofar as you described it, has always been one of principal or head teacher, and that you have always been responsible for other people. There seems to be some conflict there.

Patient: Do you mean that I didn't accept certain things? Well, I can give you an example. For instance, I couldn't accept the fact that the staff were not paid as soon as the money had arrived. Of course, handling the financial side of things was not part of my job, I never got a penny in cash because everything went straight into the convent funds. But I couldn't understand why, once the pay had arrived, and all the staff came to me because I was the headmistress . . . and they all had children and husbands, and bills to pay and things to buy, and they would ask, 'When are we going to get paid?' And I knew that the money had already arrived, and I had to make up all sorts of excuses as to why they couldn't get paid yet, but really the only reason was some clerical holdup. That was typical. In a way I was forced to be very strict with the staff, and I couldn't be, because I had built up a very good relationship with them, and with the pupils too, so this would cause a lot of friction.

I did appreciate many things though, and managed to achieve much that was good and beautiful, which gave me a great deal of satisfaction, and which I like to think back on even now. Perhaps that's what caused the trouble in the convent – someone saw that I was satisfied and successful and felt annoyed and decided to make trouble for me. That often happened. Whenever I did something worthwhile, or achieved something or got someone in the school to do something, someone in the Sisterhood always seemed to do or say something against me and then I would think, 'I just can't go on like this'.

Dr Detinis: You said that sometimes you have pains when something goes wrong at work. Were you referring to this business with the money?

Patient: No, that was before then. Now I work as a secretary; if for example something has to be done by the end of the month, then I like all the figures and so on to be ready by the 26th or 27th so that it can all be dealt with in plenty of time. And when the staff who help me with these various tasks, who have to look up facts or dates or whatever, when they don't do their jobs properly, then I feel awful. But it's this tremendous sense of responsibility that one has . . . it's too much . . . I think that things . . . I think that that's what caused all the suffering in the convent, because I believe that it's possible to work things out without hurting anybody's feelings; on the contrary, if everyone is happy then things get done properly.

Dr Detinis: Were there conflicts for these reasons?
Patient: There still are sometimes.

Dr Detinis: Arguments?
Patient: Arguments too. I sometimes try to leave things to my

husband, who's the headmaster of the school. I'm the school secretary, not his personal secretary; and sometimes when I see that there are things that might cause conflict between the staff and myself I pass them on to him. Sometimes the staff feel as though unreasonable demands are being made of them, although the fact of the matter is really that they won't do their jobs properly. One way round the problem for me is to pass things over to my husband.

Dr Detinis: Can you tell me anything else about your character? What are you like, how would you define yourself?
Patient: I'm a shrew! I'm the sort of person who puts up with things and holds their tongue but once things go beyond a certain point I explode, I really do. Sometimes – no, mostly – when I react like that, because my nerves are getting to me or I feel momentarily annoyed, I regret it for the rest of the week and desperately try to make up with the person who caused me to raise my voice a bit, because I'm quite good-natured. I normally try – my husband can tell you this – I'm normally quite mild-mannered, but I get into situations where . . . I'm usually mild and gentle. I always feel for people less fortunate than myself, I'm capable of doing anything for other people. I'm telling you this because it's one of my faults, sometimes I take their problems so much to heart that it makes me ill ('Mildness' (65/II)), 'Sympathetic' (86/I)).

Dr Detinis: Please tell me more.
Patient: Well, I don't know! I have often tended sick people, nuns who were ill. Often they were suffering from cancer, they couldn't talk any longer, and for nights on end I would watch and wait with them, pressing a moist cloth to their parched lips. Then there were lay people too, mothers of teachers at the school. I would stay by their side through days and days of agony. Sometimes I gave up what I had if they needed it more than me, but I always had the support of my husband because he's just like that too. For example, when my friends had financial problems I would always give them a little basketful of things to tide them over till the end of the month.

Dr Detinis: And are you moved by anything else regarding people whom you don't personally know?
Patient: Oh, yes, the suffering of humanity, all the trials and tribulations that our brothers and sisters go through . . . just one look at a newspaper makes me feel ill. One feels so helpless because there is nothing one can do about these things. I'm sensitive to all these things,

I think one should sometimes just let things be, otherwise one's life is full of these conflicts.

Dr Detinis: What do you mean?
Patient: Well, obviously, I sometimes feel that it might be better if I could be a bit more indifferent. They say that one has to accept things as they are.

Dr Detinis: What else can you tell me about your character?
Patient: I don't like dishonesty, I can't bear it when people lie to me! It happens to me at work, not with my husband, I work at another school too. And one sees so many things. I'm the secretary at the other school too and a lot of paperwork passes across my desk. Sometimes I've prepared a document and I ask someone to despatch it, and then I ask them again ten days later whether it went off, and they say, yes, of course it did, and three or four days later I open a cupboard and see that it's still there . . . That really annoys me, I can't stand people who are dishonest or unfair, people who preach at you and tell you endless things about justice and charity but who behave in a different way altogether ('Indignation').

Dr Detinis: Are you a loving person?
Patient: Yes, I am. I don't have many friends – my friend in all things is my husband – but those few are friends who were there when I needed them, or when they needed me, and who came to me too in times of joy. I don't see much of them because our work doesn't leave us much time to socialise. We're at school all day and we get back home late at night and on Saturdays and Sundays there are meetings and functions at the school and things to do round the house, so . . .

Dr Detinis: Is your wife a loving person?
Husband: My wife is very loving and gentle, she has been very sweet to me recently. She always tries to make me feel happy and cared for. When I buy a tie, or a shirt, or a pair of trousers, she keeps them in perfect order. She likes me to look smart, at school she always stands up for me and gets worried if there's any problems with the staff or pupils. I think it's precisely out of concern for me that she gets upset about things of no importance in our relationship. She is very affectionate, and spoils me no end.

Dr Detinis: And what are you like with children?
Patient: I love children too, and I say that because I used to teach them in nursery, primary and secondary schools. I also taught Spanish language and literature at the evening classes for adults, and that was very

nice too. I used to enjoy it so much, but there came a point about five years ago when I suddenly felt quite exhausted. I was working morning, noon and night, and my voice was quite hoarse, and I used to get home at a quarter to twelve, and I could hardly talk. It went on and on, I had to keep on working because I couldn't just stop, and finally I told myself I couldn't take it any more. I was losing my voice because I used to talk to the children so much. But I have lovely memories of them, and of the toddlers in the nursery school. I think I got rather worn out and it didn't do my throat any good at all.

Dr Detinis: And were you affectionate with the children?
Patient: Yes, I was.

Dr Detinis: There are many ways of showing affection.
Patient: Yes, but I used to take an interest in them, help them . . . As a nun I taught religious education and ethics, and I talked to the girls with a great deal of love and they treated me in the same way. They would ask me things, ask my advice. I always cared about them and always wanted to give them more of myself.

Dr Detinis: Do you have any fears?
Patient: I'm always afraid! Not of being widowed but . . . I'm always scared that something will happen to my husband or to myself; we are so happy, and God has given us so much in these five years that I think we are blessed with too many things. We have good jobs, we love each other very much, we help each other all the time; he is always concerned about my health and I for his, so I think this fear about it all coming to an end . . . It's not that I distrust him in the slightest, because really the only thing I believe in is my husband . . .

Dr Detinis: Do you have any other, more specific fears?
Patient: At one time I was scared of losing my job, but not any more. There wasn't much job security in the private schools where I worked after leaving the convent, and the Fathers were terribly capricious and sometimes gave you work and then took it all away again ('Anxiety, future, about' (7/I)).

Dr Detinis: You said at one point that one of the things that distressed you most was when your aunt told you there was no money left. And now you just mentioned your fear of losing your job. How do you feel your situation as it is now?
Patient: If I lost my job, I wouldn't be able to find another one at my age and in my state of health. I have never done anything else except teach. I think that when I retire, I'll look for something to do, I'll find

something because I don't want to be completely idle. But teaching is what I'm best at.

Dr Detinis: Your husband said that you once lived in poverty. Are you scared of doing so again?
Patient: No, I'm not scared of that. That's why I said that God has given us so much. When I left the convent I didn't own anything, not even a single piece of furniture in the room where I was living.

Dr Detinis: Do you have any other fears – such as, for example, a fear of storms or the dark?
Patient: Yes, storms, and the wind . . .

Dr Detinis: Why?
Patient: I don't know how to put it. We used to have a house on the coast at Reta – we've sold it now – it's a beautiful place with wonderful beaches. It was very windy though, and the first two years we spent the summer there I felt very ill, because of the wind . . . it made me very nervous, very jittery.

Dr Detinis: The wind or the storms?
Patient: Both.

Dr Detinis: Are you scared of storms here?
Patient: No.

Dr Detinis: Do you have any fears when you're alone?
Patient: Yes, I just want him to come home quickly.

Dr Detinis: Are you scared of heights, of enclosed places? Of thieves, animals, dogs . . . ?
Patient: I'm scared of dogs, but that's because they've attacked me so many times.

Dr Detinis: And before they attacked you were you scared of them?
Patient: I can't remember. When I see a dog I have to cross the street.

Dr Detinis: Puppies too?
Patient: No, not puppies, just dogs. I think that dogs know I'm scared of them because when I cross the street they come after me.

Dr Detinis: Are you scared of illnesses?
Patient: Just this arthritis of mine – of being disabled.

Dr Detinis: But not of other illnesses?
Patient: No.

Dr Detinis: Of death?
Patient: Yes, I'm very scared of death, but it's because I want to live. I

was already grown up when I married and I want to enjoy the company of my husband, we're so happy that death seems . . .

Dr Detinis: Before you married, were you scared of death?
Patient: No.

Dr Detinis: Are you a tidy person?
Patient: Yes. I put my things . . . Sometimes the lady who comes to clean moves them and I . . . I like to keep things in their proper place . . . I keep everything in order.

Dr Detinis: What effect does the weather have on you?
Patient: Up to about two or three years ago I used to be very sensitive to the cold and didn't like it at all, but that's all changed now.

Dr Detinis: Can you tolerate hot weather?
Patient: Yes, I can.

Dr Detinis: The sun?
Patient: The sun no, I hardly ever sunbathe because I can't take it; it hurts my eyes.

Dr Detinis: Can you go out when it's sunny?
Patient: Yes, that's alright, it doesn't bother me.

Dr Detinis: Do you like the sea climate?
Patient: It's not good for me, that's where the problems with my hip started . . . ('Generalities, air, seashore' (1344/II)).

Dr Detinis: Does any kind of clothing bother you?
Patient: No.

Dr Detinis: On what parts of your body do you perspire?
Patient: My perspiration is normal, I only perspire under the armpits.

Dr Detinis: What's your favourite food?
Patient: Oh, I'm very greedy! Sweet things . . . and roasts! ('Desires sweets' (486/II))

Dr Detinis: Do you like animal fat?
Patient: No, I can't stand fat; I only use a drop of oil when I cook; I've got used to cooking without oil or fat.

Dr Detinis: Bitter or sour things?
Patient: I like grapefruit.

Dr Detinis: Spicy things?
Patient: Oh, yes!

Dr Detinis: Hot things?
Patient: A pickled meat dish, properly prepared. I use lots of spices.

Dr Detinis: Milk?
Patient: I like milk too; creamy dishes, custard . . .

Dr Detinis: At what temperature do you like your food and drink?
Patient: There are some things I can't eat if they're cold, usually. I like them hot, but not too hot.

Dr Detinis: Do you have periods?
Patient: Not any more, Doctor. I began to have problems when I was forty-five and it's nearly a year since . . .

Dr Detinis: Was there anything about your periods which seemed unusual?
Patient: No.

Dr Detinis: Did your character change in any way at that time of the month?
Patient: The pains in my bones were worse, and quite often I would get into a tizz about things . . .

Dr Detinis: How did you feel?
Patient: Rather depressed, and I sometimes had terrible migraines and had to go and lie down . . . before the period.

Dr Detinis: Do you normally sleep well?
Patient: Yes, but I don't sleep long enough.

Dr Detinis: Do you wake up easily in the morning?
Patient: Yes, Doctor.

Dr Detinis: In what position do you sleep?
Patient: Always on my side.

Dr Detinis: On either side?
Patient: No, always on the right-hand side. I could never sleep on my left-hand side.

Dr Detinis: Why not?
Patient: I don't like it, I don't feel comfortable. I feel as though my breathing is more . . . ('Generalities, lying, side, on, left, agg.' (1373/I)).

Dr Detinis: You mentioned your dreams . . .
Patient: Yes, I told you that I often had the same dream. And I also used to dream that all my teeth were falling out and that when I put my hand up to my mouth I would be holding all my teeth in my hand. But I don't any more . . . ('Sleep, dreams, teeth, breaking off, falling out, pulled out' (1243/II)).

185

Dr Detinis: When was that?

Patient: When I was at the convent. It was always the same dream that I had over and over again, like a nightmare.

Dr Detinis: Did you have any other dream?

Patient: Yes, I wanted to go somewhere and I either didn't have one of my stockings or I was coming down the stairs, I was always going somewhere.

Dr Detinis: You said that you bottle things up until you explode, and then you go and look for the person who made you lose your temper, and talk to them. Why do you do that?

Patient: I worry that when I'm rude to someone because of my nerves, I might have offended them, or hurt their feelings, and I could have put it more gently . . .

Dr Detinis: What do you feel?

Patient: I get upset and so I try to start talking to them to show that there are no hard feelings.

Dr Detinis: Is there someone with whom you get on very badly, or have done in the past?

Patient: There's a school employee who is a great effort to put up with. She's the sort of person who likes to come and . . . She doesn't annoy me . . . She's someone, bless her, who probably means well, but . . . she's a terrible gossip . . . When one works in the school office there are many things that have to be kept confidential – I know that people have talked openly about private matters outside the school, I know that that it was her and I get very annoyed.

COMMENTARY

I encouraged the patient to continue her lengthy but spontaneous account for as long as she did, because the case is an extremely interesting one. There are many characteristic symptoms, but beyond this, what we saw was a history of successive emotional frustrations. She wasn't loved by her mother, who sent her to live with her aunt. Her aunt put her in a boarding school. She hoped to find love and security in the convent. Then she writes to her mother in Villa Maria, telling her that she is shortly to take the veil, but gets no reply. She was trying to re-establish contact with her mother: once more, she was seeking love and affection. Later she said, 'I regret not having had a normal relationship with my sister, I love her very much, but the convent separated us, drew us apart.' She fears she may lose the love she has found. When she gets angry with someone, she regrets it and tries 'desperately' to effect a reconciliation, because, as she said, she is 'very loving'. Her husband told us, 'She tries to make me feel happy . . . she spoils me no end.'

She really is as gentle as she says she is. This is evident from her attitude, her gestures and her tone of voice.

REPERTORISATION

'Anxiety, conscience, of, (as if guilty of a crime)' (6/I)
'Anxiety, future, about' (7/I)
'Fear, happen, something will' (45/II)
'Desires sweets' (486/II)
'Mildness' (65/II)
'Generalities, air, seashore' (1344/II)
'Dreams, teeth, falling out, breaking off, pulled out' (1243/II)
'Lying, side, on, left, agg.' (1373/I)
'Pain, wandering' (1389/II)

Prescription: Natrum Muriaticum 1M.

FOLLOW-UP

(*Seven months after the first prescription*)

For ten days after taking the remedy, Mrs E. had an intense aggravation of her rheumatic pains, this time in all her joints at the same time. There then followed an almost complete amelioration of the pains. A sore throat, from which she had not suffered for three years, and constipation, which she had not had for two years, returned in reverse order of appearance. She also began menstruating again one year after the start of her treatment. Her migraines, the tension in her neck and the hot flushes also disappeared. She felt calmer and more optimistic. All her presenting symptoms improved. Over a further two years of treatment, she received ascending potencies of Natrum Muriaticum up to CM on the centesimal scale and 12 on the LM scale.

Case V: Maria P., aged 28, single

Dr Detinis: Tell me what you would like to discuss.

Patient: I have been taking homoeopathic remedies for about two years. I went to a homoeopath because of a problem with my nerves. I was on 3mg of Lexotan (benzodiazepine) three times a day.

Dr Detinis: What symptoms do you have?

Patient: Well, the symptoms seem to have become less acute. I used to get strong spasms in my cervix and my back; my nerves were very bad and I got headaches. After that I had problems with my bowels, with my sight, and irregular periods. The bowel problems seem to be related to my work. I'm a teacher, and during the school year I'm rather tense and nervous, and that's when I get them, but now, during the holidays, I don't. I teach Physical Education. Those are the symptoms I had, in fact I've still got them.

I've come to see you now because I wanted to ask about some medication I was given when I hurt my leg while I was on holiday. I had out-patients treatment and they prescribed Cicatrin (an anti-bacterial). When I got back to Buenos Aires I had a sort of rash all over my body and I wondered whether it was a reaction to the Cicatrin. That seemed to give me a bout of flu which laid me up for three weeks.

Just before that I had taken a follow-up dose of Ignatia, and nothing happened, it had no effect at all. But now I'm not sure whether it had a delayed effect which caused the rash and the flu. It really wiped me out. I wanted to ask if there is something I could take for things like that, whether there's a homoeopathic equivalent to antibiotics. Or, for instance, is there anything I could take when I get a head-cold and can't sleep?

Dr Detinis: Can you remember what potency the Ignatia was?

Patient: No . . . it was a low one.

Dr Detinis: How do you feel apart from that?

Patient: At the moment I feel as though the treatment isn't really helping, but of course the outlook is bleak as far as work is concerned at the moment. No one in arts-related subjects really knows whether they'll have a job next year because there just aren't many contracts to be had. So I've been feeling more and more tense and insecure and anxious.

Now I'm taking up a new post and everything seems to be coming back, the spasms, the stress and the fatigue. I used to get home at six in the evening feeling completely worn out; I could barely drag myself home. After a few hours I'd feel a bit better, but at first I was quite exhausted. I'm worried about that, and also about all the stress at work. It's going to be a problem until I settle in a bit at the new school. But what I'm really worried about is the tiredness; I was totally exhausted by the end of the last school year. It's partly due to the fact that I only graduated recently and I only started teaching last year, so I'm still quite inexperienced and the work takes up a lot of energy. I teach at two primary schools, to about eight groups of children in each one. And like I said, it's the exhaustion I felt that really worries me. For a start, teachers don't stop working at the end of the school day; you have to prepare things, read a lot . . . The minute I sit down at my desk in the evening I fall asleep over my books. I find it very hard to think straight, sometimes I have to read a passage two or three times in order to take it in, which I don't normally have to do. I'm really worried about being so exhausted; on Mondays I'm already tired and by Tuesday I'm just dragging myself along. I have an evening class on Tuesdays and it's all I can do to stay awake through that.

Dr Detinis: What do you think is the cause of all this exhaustion?
Patient: Well, I think that at the moment it's my relative lack of experience of working with children. And everything is so hectic in Buenos Aires; I commute in and have to rush from one school to the other. I leave home in the morning and only get back at night . . . that must have a lot to do with it. Once or twice a week I have to come into the centre of town and then I return home exhausted; all those traffic jams, all the cars honking their horns . . . It takes a huge effort just to travel on the bus, but really even that doesn't explain why I should feel so tired, though I . . . I find it easier to get through two consecutive dance classes than to have to change buses two or three times.

Dr Detinis: I would like you to go into more detail about all of this.
Patient: Well, as I said, it's about a year and a half since I graduated. For a start, higher education in some colleges in Buenos Aires is not very good. Then you have to find work and you hope to be able to fill in the gaps in the course of time, but there just isn't the time to do that. The whole system is wrong, it's not just higher education. So all this lack of theoretical support makes me feel very insecure, not about the work itself, because I think I'm quite capable, but on the practical side, it's difficult to set the right standards for the children. And then I get more and more tense and arrive at school in a terrible state after having had to change buses twice on the way . . . I arrive worrying about

whether what I've prepared will be interesting or not . . . I find it hard to cope with everything that crops up during the day.

Dr Detinis: You've had these symptoms for two years?

Patient: Yes, for quite a long time. When I was a student I used to worry what would become of me after I graduated. I wasn't sure if I was doing the right course, I worried about whether I would be able to find work. There was a big question mark over my future: what was I going to do with my degree?

Dr Detinis: You mean as regards getting a job?

Patient: Yes, exactly.

Dr Detinis: And when did all these symptoms appear? The spasms, the headaches, problems with your bowels . . .

Patient: Well, for years . . . I couldn't put a date to it because I've had them for quite a while now. Half way through college I changed courses.

Dr Detinis: From what?

Patient: History of art.

Dr Detinis: Why did you drop that?

Patient: Because it was taking too long, it was quite difficult, and it's very hard to find work with that kind of a degree. I'm still interested in it – I'd like to take it up again some time, but as a personal thing. What I'm doing now is quite closely related to it.

I suppose my problems began when I was about eighteen. I began to lose weight . . . Then I was treated for some kind of crisis – crying fits. I was on a surgery auxiliary course at the hospital and I couldn't cope with the environment there. At about that time I started to have fainting fits – I'm not really sure what to call them. I didn't exactly faint, I just couldn't talk or see anything, though I could still hear things. I couldn't control my body, That happened two or three times over five years or so, till I was twenty-three. I had neurological treatment, I was taking . . . the last thing I took was some tranquillisers, which made me feel very bad. I was walking around like a zombie, so I decided it was best to stop taking it. I changed neurologists and that's when I began to take Lexotan. I didn't have any problems with that except for a lot of muscular fatigue. I was on Lexotan for quite a long time, but I was worried about the fact that I was dependent on it and was having to take more and more of it. At first it was one tablet, then two and finally three or even four.

Dr Detinis: What did you say you couldn't cope with?

Patient: The fact that I was in a hospital. I couldn't stand the contact with the patients, seeing them in pain and not being able to help.

Something quite funny happened once; we were learning how to apply sterile dressings to a patient who was in a lot of pain, and I was feeling really ill. I turned round to my friend, who was about to apply a dressing, and said, 'Just blow on it!' – which of course is the one thing you shouldn't do.

So obviously I was deeply affected by all the suffering, and I also felt very strongly about the fact that the patients were treated as objects ('Indignation' (55/I)).

Dr Detinis: Did you do anything?

Patient: Well, at first I wanted to drop the course. I couldn't just start shouting at the doctors and nurses so I kept quiet and got more and more tense. I had terrible spasms in my jaw . . . Then I had eczema and so on.

Dr Detinis: Your attitude towards the way in which patients were being treated says a lot about you. I would like you to go into more detail about that side of your personality.

Patient: Essentially it comes down to two things: I can't stand any form of injustice or disrespect ('Indignation'). That's what's wrong with this country now, it's the same in teaching here in Buenos Aires. The situation is awful. One of the schools is in a deprived area where conditions are really tough. That kind of thing makes me really angry.

Dr Detinis: You said something about seeing patients in pain. Could you expand on that?

Patient: I wish there was a machine that could measure pain. I feel so helpless when I know that there are people in pain – patients in the hospital – and I can't do anything to help, to make the pain go away.

Dr Detinis: Do you mean physical pain specifically?

Patient: No, not just that. Physical pain because it's something very concrete, but you can feel emotional pain too. Above all I feel bad that there are no fast-acting cures. Part of the reason for that must be my anxiety, wanting to have everything now. I can see, for instance, that children need time to learn how things work, just as adults need time to learn to live in a democracy . . . I find it very hard to be patient, I get very anxious.

Dr Detinis: You said you were sensitive, could you give us some examples?

Patient: Well, I'm very weepy, very emotional. Mind you I've only let myself cry, particularly in front of other people, for the last two years or so.

Dr Detinis: What were you like before? Why did you change?

Patient: I don't really know, because it was part of a process. Being able to express myself . . . I think it's got something to do with the way I was brought up. If I felt happy or unhappy I couldn't show it. I wasn't allowed to – if I did they would disapprove. So I learnt to hide my feelings, repress them. Recently I've started to let go a bit and I feel a lot better. So now if I hear or see something that makes me want to cry, well then I do.

Dr Detinis: And what if there are people watching you?

Patient: I feel rather embarrassed but I carry on.

Dr Detinis: And if they try to console you?

Patient: Sometimes it makes me feel better and sometimes it doesn't, but I couldn't say in what circumstances.

Dr Detinis: You said that between the ages of eighteen and twenty-three you had fainting fits. What exactly were they like, how long did they last?

Patient: They were the ones I already told you about. It felt as though I suddenly had a short circuit, or as though I unplugged myself, my eyes shut tight . . . ('Faintness, hysterical' (1360/I)). I don't think I collapsed, because I could choose a place to sit down, that kind of thing. It was as if I was experiencing a terrible kind of reality and I wanted to unplug myself and let go. It happened two or three times, they used to last about half an hour and then I'd slowly come round.

Dr Detinis: Do you remember on what occasions this happened?

Patient: The first time I was still at secondary school, in the sixth form. The second time I was at the hospital, and the last one I can't remember . . . I think that again it was a quiet moment, when I could just let myself go. It was as though I suddenly became aware and thought, 'Right, I want to get out of here.' And once I lost consciousness when I knocked my elbow on something, I just fainted away. They took me to hospital . . . because it happened in the street. That's when I started having neurological treatment.

Dr Detinis: Was it due to some crisis, watching an operation or something like that?

Patient: No, not then, but afterwards. It happened in very tense situations. Once there was a break-in and a gunfight at the university and while it was going on I could act, move, help a friend . . . And then

192

when it was all over I could cry . . . but not till then.

Dr Detinis: Where do you live?

Patient: With my parents.

Dr Detinis: Have you got brothers and sisters?

Patient: No.

Dr Detinis: Have you got a steady boyfriend?

Patient: No!

Dr Detinis: Have you had one?

Patient: Once, for a short time. It was a very important relationship and I still haven't managed to get over it.

Dr Detinis: Can you tell me about it?

Patient: It happened four years ago. After a while we decided . . . that we didn't love each other . . . But then I realized that I did still love him.

Dr Detinis: And did that affect you in any way?

Patient: Oh, yes. For quite a long time I felt very upset, very sad, I didn't want to see anybody . . . I carried on with my life, working and studying, but I became very withdrawn, I didn't see much of other people.

Dr Detinis: Do you have any memories from your childhood?

Patient: Well, there was a time when my parents didn't get on together; that's how it seemed, anyway. But they didn't separate, and now they get on very well. I seem to have a different image of it now.

Dr Detinis: Can you remember what you were like as a child?

Patient: I'm told I was a very good little girl, but I didn't like being like that . . . hah, you have to be very good. But when I was older that began to annoy me and I started to rebel . . . I turned against my parents. But I think that's a natural part of adolescence, wanting your independence, your own life . . . I get on well with my parents now.

Dr Detinis: What's life like now?

Patient: My life now? The children, work . . . I spent such a long time working as a temp, always working in different places, and now I'm doing something I enjoy . . . My parents, well . . . since I live with them . . . we talk a lot; and then there are my friends. And well, there are lots of things I'd like to do.

Dr Detinis: Such as?

Patient: I'd like to have more time to study, more time to go out, to go to classes, more time to do nothing at all, which can be a real luxury sometimes, more time to make things, but . . .

Dr Detinis: When you say 'do nothing', what do you mean?
Patient: Well, literally, just to stare at the ceiling, have time to sit and think . . . or to do things around the house. I don't mind doing housework, as long as I'm not in a hurry or don't feel obliged to do it. Lots of things, really. I'd like to have more time to read, for instance. There are some books I have to get through for Tuesday, and I'd rather be able to take more time over them, but . . .

Dr Detinis: Do you mean to say that you need time to do things?
Patient: Yes, I'm very slow; I need time to think things over, to reflect . . . And I also need time to do things. The nicest thing about holidays is getting up and having a quiet cup of tea, I don't even read the paper . . . and I can't do that now. I'm slow because I hate to hurry. My natural pace is slow and gentle . . . I'm not always like that, though, because when I'm dancing, for example, I can speed up in time to the music without any trouble. But normally I do things very slowly ('Slowness' (81/I)).

Dr Detinis: Things like eating, walking . . . Does this ever cause problems?
Patient: Yes, all the time.

Dr Detinis: I should like to go back to something you mentioned earlier, something that happened when you were eighteen. Could you tell us about that?
Patient: It was a very difficult time for me. By and large I've got over it now, but it still hurts to think back on it.

Dr Detinis: How would you sum it up?
Patient: I suppose I went through a phase, a crisis. I was very mixed up.

Dr Detinis: What was the problem?
Patient: Around that time there was quite a traumatic change in my life – I changed schools. I spent three years at a very nice secondary school with a fairly small intake of pupils, where the relationship with the teachers was very good, a one-to-one relationship. And then I changed schools, I went to a very large school where I was just a number rather than a person and that obviously affected me profoundly. I was on a Business Studies course and didn't like it at all, it just didn't interest me. It was family pressure, really, that made me do it. And it had a profound effect on me.

194

Case V: Maria P., aged 28, single

Dr Detinis: You became 'just a number rather than a person' . . . how would you define that?
Patient: Well, you see, the primary school and my first secondary school were like an extension of my family. Moving to a school where there were lots of other people around came as a pretty rude shock. That's what it came down to. I felt like a piece of furniture or a machine . . . I found my course very boring and just couldn't motivate myself to learn everything I had to.

Oh, there's something else I wanted to say about rhythms. I've often noticed – this is a little theory I have – that when I'm with people who have a different rhythm to me, a much faster one, I seem to identify with them, and when I'm with people whose rhythm is slower than mine, I speed up. Perhaps its got something to do with equilibrium or compensation. When I was studying, I had a friend with a much faster rhythm than me, which was good for some things, but not so good for others. So we sort of balanced each other out.

Dr Detinis: Do you adapt yourself to other people?
Patient: Yes, I try to, when I'm working or studying with people I don't have anything in common with.

Dr Detinis: Are you a loving person?
Patient: Yes I am, I take to people immediately and then quite often I have to distance myself from them a bit, if I see certain things I don't like. I give myself completely, I'm completely honest and sincere, and of course people don't always respond like that. Then I have to try and restrain all my emotions, and that can be hard. I keep telling myself not to be so stupid, to keep a grip on myself and not get so involved, but . . . At the beginning it's me who gives rather than takes, I let the other person get to know me before I get to know them. Sometimes it works out, and sometimes it doesn't. And when it doesn't I back off and feel angry, angry that there's no response, angry that I've been deceived ('Love, ailments, from disappointed' (63/II)).

Dr Detinis: Why do you feel deceived?
Patient: I feel as though my trust has been abused. I start by assuming that everyone is worthy of trust, although of course not everyone is. It's the same when I realise that people aren't always completely honest, perhaps without really meaning to be . . . I don't always become angry, it's just that from then on there's something missing in the relationship, or it starts to break up – of course I'm talking about relationships with men as well as about friendships. Sometimes things

patch themselves up, but not always. I never get really annoyed with anyone; it soon blows over.

Dr Detinis: Could you tell us briefly about your character, what you're like?

Patient: That's hard to do in a few words. It's as though my personality is essentially open to a lot of possibilities – it isn't rigid or stable. Everything affects me, nothing passes me by, for better or worse. Whether I'm sad or cheerful, I'm indifferent to nothing ('Sensitive, oversensitive' (78/II)). And I'm a conciliator, I try to bring people together. That's true of my work and studies, as well as in relationships in general. In group situations it's always me who's the level-headed one with the good advice.

Dr Detinis: Do you mean in your relationship with others, or as regards other people's relationships?

Patient: Ordinary relationships with one or more people . . .

Dr Detinis: And what do the others think of you?

Patient: I think they see me as a conciliator.

Dr Detinis: Are you afraid of anything?

Patient: It's hard to say now – there seem to have been a lot of changes recently. My fears used to relate to what I was doing; whether or not I would be able to succeed. My greatest fear when I was studying was of having to confront pupils, children, having to be a teacher. To some extent that fear is still there ('Confidence, want of self' (13/II)).

Dr Detinis: Do you have any other fears? For example of heights, enclosed places . . . ?

Patient: I wouldn't really call it a fear, but, yes, of very enclosed spaces.

Dr Detinis: Of using a lift?

Patient: No.

Dr Detinis: How do you feel when you're alone?

Patient: Well, I get bored of being alone and look for company, but I'm not scared.

Dr Detinis: Are you scared of burglars, thunderstorms . . . death?

Patient: Well . . . I'm still quite young so I don't worry about that too much.

Dr Detinis: You said that you were sensitive, that things affect you strongly. What things affect you or move you most?

Patient: Anger and fury . . . and injustice, I feel very strongly about that. ('Indignation'). I'm also very sentimental, I have a feeling for poems and songs . . . certain places, certain memories. There's one particular childhood memory of the countryside. Whenever I catch the smell of wood-smoke it all comes flooding back.

Dr Detinis: Do you feel moved by Nature?

Patient: Oh yes – by the sea, and in the mountains. The sea most of all. Mind you, it takes me a few days to get used to it.

Dr Detinis: In what circumstances do you feel jealous?

Patient: Well, let me give you a couple of examples. For instance, I was the only girl in the whole family and I don't think I would have liked having any other cousins. And then when my most important relationship ended because of another woman, that made me very angry too.

Dr Detinis: How tidy are you?

Patient: I used to be very tidy. I like being tidy, but now I don't worry about it too much because I just don't have the time.

Dr Detinis: How well do you sleep?

Patient: Usually well, except when I'm feeling tense because of something I have to do the next day, and then I keep waking up . . . I often feel very tired when I wake up. Now that I've started working again I wake up feeling exhausted.

Dr Detinis: In what position do you sleep?

Patient: On my side; usually I go to sleep on my left-hand side and then change to the right-hand side.

Dr Detinis: Do you have a recurring dream?

Patient: Different things happen to my teeth – they break or fall out.

Dr Detinis: What are your periods like?

Patient: Pretty irregular, they tend to be very early and sometimes they are very heavy. They last five or six days.

Dr Detinis: How do you feel before, during and after your periods?

Patient: Very occasionally I know when my periods are coming. When they start I feel slightly giddy.

Dr Detinis: What effect does the weather have on you?

Patient: I don't like damp weather, it makes me retain fluids.

Dr Detinis: How do you feel right now?

Patient: When I was in the waiting room I felt as though I was about to take an exam, because of the other people here. I felt as though I was being talked about. It was quite unpleasant, like being trapped. I do confide in certain people, and I don't necessarily need to have known them for long – it's the quality of the relationship that counts – and then I'll talk about myself freely.

Dr Detinis: How did you feel before taking exams?

Patient: Awful! I always used to get very bad marks at university because I was scared out of my wits in oral exams and couldn't say anything . . . my mind would just go blank. And my feet felt strange, as though they would disappear into the ground. ('Anticipation, complaints from' (4/I)).

Dr Detinis: You don't like the damp; what else is bad for you?

Patient: I don't like extreme heat and cold or dryness and dampness . . . I don't like extremes of any kind. The sun is bad for me, the combination of sun and sea gives me a kind of rash or allergy, with very strong itching . . .

Dr Detinis: How do you feel in the wind, in cloudy weather, in storms?

Patient: I like storms and cloudy weather, and the sun too, but I can't take too much of it, otherwise I get a headache and feel ill. I like cloudy weather.

Dr Detinis: Do you wear woollen clothes?

Patient: Never against my skin, I can't stand it.

Dr Detinis: Do you mind if my colleagues ask you a few more questions?

Patient: Of course not.

QUESTIONS FROM THE FLOOR

Question: What sort of food do you like?

Patient: Sweet things on the whole, and anything salty. I don't eat much meat, and I like vegetables. I quite like fruit.

Question: How did your parents get on together?

Patient: They didn't get on too well for a while, I don't remember exactly because I was very young. They used to row and fight.

Question: Can you remember how you felt then?

Patient: Well, I cried, I used to run away and cry. At that time I wasn't really allowed to cry in public, or laugh too much, or feel happy. There were problems with money.

Question: What were your mother and father like as people – how would you define them?

Patient: My mother is in charge at home. She seems to be the one who takes decisions, although they discuss things together. My father's used to it. Mother takes the practical decisions, so to speak, and he takes the more emotional ones, do you see what I mean? He has a bit more of a say in family matters.

Question: How did you feel in this family situation?

Patient: Well, it was different at different times. When I was a little girl I was the centre of attention because I was the only child, and when I was a teenager it was the same, but then everyone seemed to be criticising me. And now I feel as though I were almost a parent to them. All three of us sit down and talk things over.

Question: Are there any aspects of your personality which you have had all through your life?

Patient: Yes, I think so, but as they seemed negative, I tried to change them. I learned to keep quiet, for instance, instead of objecting or protesting and trying to change things. There are things that make me very angry and which I'm always questioning, but there's another part of me which says, 'No, keep quiet'.

Question: How do you get on with your mother at the moment?

Patient: At the moment we don't get on too well, we quarrel a lot. When I was in my teens I ran away from home. But now that we're all older we seem to be able to accept each other. It's as though I'm more or less aware of what's happening to her and she knows what's happening to me.

Question: Would you say that there was more acceptance than affection?

Patient: No, no.

Question: I wanted to ask you if you felt that you had reconciled your parents to each other and that it was because of you that they didn't separate.

Patient: No, I think it was their decision. I don't think they ever really intended to separate because their outlook is very traditional and conservative. Anyway, I don't think it had anything to do with me.

Question: What are you like with money?

Patient: I'm terrible! When I get paid and I have all that money in front of me I think I'm rich and I let myself spend it and then at the end of the month . . . Oh, one thing more about illnesses: I easily get a temperature or problems with my skin, but very rarely get infections.

COMMENTARY

What do you think are the most salient and important aspects of the personality of this woman, which are the characteristic symptoms that will lead us to her constitutional remedy?

Well, first of all, there is her obvious insecurity, which in the terms of the *Repertory* is 'Confidence, want of self' (13/II) and 'Anticipation, complaints from' (4/I) – in this case, before examinations.

The patient probably had a repressive upbringing; she was not allowed to do many things. Only in recent years could she let herself cry in front of other people. Everything she told us about is a symptom from a remedy, so why have I emphasised this business of her crying? Well, some remedies do not cry in the presence of others, some cry when they do not want to and cannot cry when they want to. Natrum Muriaticum, for example, never cries in public. This is a repressed patient.

There are no obvious conflicts in her relationship with her parents. Of the mental symptoms, the most important one is how the patient behaves emotionally, how loving she is. Some remedies are less likely to have problems on the emotional level, such as Calcarea Carbonica and Sulphur and many others. In this case, however, there is nothing about the patient's emotional state which can be translated into the terms of the materia medica or the repertory.

One of this woman's most important characteristics is her hypersensitivity, which she revealed in several ways. When asked what was the most important aspect of her personality she paused and replied, 'Everything affects me, nothing passes me by, for better or worse, I'm indifferent to nothing'. And her account revealed her sensitivity to the suffering of the patients in the hospital when she was there on a course. She is affected by suffering and sadness. She is hypersensitive to moral and emotional impressions.

As a child she was very likeable, the centre of attention, all the more so as she was an only child; at school she didn't want to be 'just a number' and suffered as a result. This patient almost certainly has hysterical traits. Her convulsions were badly treated by one doctor. The second neurologist noticed this, and put her on a tranquilliser. The fainting fits were typically hysterical; she 'chose a place to sit down', and she wanted to 'unplug' herself. This is another general symptom: 'Faintness, hysterical' (1360/I). The desire to be the centre of attention, the star of the show, is typically hysterical. The patient's behaviour, the way she came in and sat down, her way of talking, was that of someone who is acting, who, despite her inhibitions, is an artist in life.

The patient said she feels very strongly about disrespect and injustice. The *Synthetic Repertory* has the rubric 'Injustice, cannot support' (column 633), which concerns ethical aspects of the personality. It contains only three remedies, but the symptom is covered by a much broader heading in Kent: 'Indignation' (55/II).

'Slowness' (81/I) is another symptom.

Homoeopaths are liable to get very excited when a patient tells them that they dream their teeth are breaking or falling out. When very few remedies cover a given symptom which is highly characteristic and attractive, but which does not match the totality of the case, then it must be ignored. A key symptom is one that reveals the true nature of the case; but it must always fit in with everything else. Natrum Muriaticum and Nux Vomica both have this symptom in different ways. However, the patient does not have the characteristic symptoms of either of these remedies.

One might next take the symptom 'Sympathetic' (86/I), meaning compassionate. Great care must be taken here because we must be confident that the symptom is always present, and not just in situations where the patient is identifying with the suffering of another person. Compassion may be expressed actively or passively; a person may be sympathetic without necessarily acting to help the person who is suffering.

Impatience is another symptom, a characteristic of the hysterical person who wants everything now. It is related to anxiety.

The patient was deeply affected when her boyfriend left her. She told us that she was very upset for a long time afterwards. She is loving, gets on well with her friends and misses them when they are not there. She said that she lets people get to know her before she gets to know them, and ultimately has to 'back off' from them. She grieves and suffers when she is separated from people, and when she is deceived. This symptom is 'Love, ailments, from disappointed' (63/II). (The reader will see that I have nevertheless not repertorised this symptom. In the event, it came through less strongly than the five rubrics that were selected.)

This characteristic, together with her great hypersensibility to moral impressions, leads me to believe that her constitutional remedy is indeed the one she has been taking for the last two years, albeit in a low potency – Ignatia. No other remedy suffers so much from parting or from unrequited love. Other remedies are also strongly indicated: Calcarea Carbonica, Natrum Muriaticum and Pulsatilla, which, together with Ignatia, is the remedy that best covers the symptomatology.

Let us establish a differential diagnosis between Ignatia and Pulsatilla, firstly with regard to one particular symptom which is very typical of both – 'Yielding', from the *Synthetic Repertory* (column 1102).

Pulsatilla yields because she is dependent, being emotionally immature, but she does not get angry and would not run away from home, as this woman did. She may leave the family home, but only to seek out a substitute, because she is always looking for substitutes. Pulsatilla never suffers from ailments from unrequited love, because she always attaches herself to paternal or maternal substitutes as a result of this emotional dependency. This is an important difference. Pulsatilla would not have behaved in the way that this woman did.

Ignatia gives in to others. When involved in a relationship her behaviour is very principled and submissive, as she fears she will lose her partner. She suffers at every parting. This is a deep and important characteristic of Ignatia. Ignatia does not, unlike Pulsatilla, feel forsaken, but she does have a fear of separation.

Ignatia is meticulous and very obsessive. Dr Candegabe has characterised it as 'the hyper-obsessive remedy of the materia medica'.

Pulsatilla is not primarily an angry remedy; it does not appear as a grade three in any of the Anger headings in the *Repertory*. The Pulsatilla patient is typically very conciliatory; she always wants everything to be alright. Although Maria says she is a conciliator, she is also a very angry person.

The rubric 'Violent' (91/II) includes many remedies, but Pulsatilla is notably absent; she is never violent or spiteful. Nor does Pulsatilla appear under 'Injustice, cannot support' (*Synthetic Repertory*, column 633).

The patient said, 'I'm very weepy, very emotional'. Pulsatilla is the cry-baby of the materia medica; she cries uninhibitedly, even in the presence of other people. As this patient is very repressed, we cannot draw conclusions about her tendency to cry. One must always see the symptom in the context of the patient's life, for this reveals whether or not it is of value.

'Confidence, want of self' (13/II) is also shared by Pulsatilla. Both remedies are slow – 'Slowness' (81/I).

Ignatia, like Lycopodium, may be domineering; Pulsatilla never is. Ignatia is frequently indicated in young women who have suffered emotional frustrations and who have this tendency to yield. In Ignatia everything is exaggerated and dramatised; she swings between extremes.

Not all hysterical cases are covered by Ignatia, nor is everything in Ignatia hysterical. This is evident from Kent's *Lectures on Homoeopathic Materia Medica*.

REPERTORISATION

'Indignation' (55/II)
'Confidence, want of self' (13/II)
'Anticipation, complaints from' (4/I)
'Slowness' (81/I)
'Faintness, hysterical' (1360/I)

Prescription: Ignatia 10M.

Case VI: Stella C., aged 29, separated, no children

Dr Detinis: Tell me what brings you here.

Patient: I haven't come about anything specific, just lots of different things. I'm very confused about everything at the moment, and very depressed too. I'm trying to sort out my life, but I just can't manage it. I don't socialise very much, and I find it hard to get on with people. I'm on a teacher training course at university but I'm not sure if it's really what I want to do. It's the same with work; I don't really feel suited to any kind of job. I just don't have the strength to face up to things. I tend to do what I think I ought to more than what I really want to do. I seem to live in a constant state of contradiction between duty and desire ('Will, contradiction of' (95/I)). I can't even think straight.

If I could, I wouldn't spend my life in the company of other people at all. I always want to run away to somewhere where there's no one at all, where there's no one to see me in this state ('Indifference, loved ones, to' (55/I)). . . . I have to face up to reality, it's as though I've only just begun to realise that I'm living in a society that makes certain demands of me. I find it terribly hard to give, because I feel as though nothing I can do is worth anything. I'm terribly passive and power-less – that's how I feel, at any rate. I can't cope with all the demands that are made of me; I always push myself but I never feel I can give enough. I don't know what else I can say.

Dr Detinis: Everything that you have said so far was very well put and extremely useful; please continue in the same way.

Patient: Well, for example, I'm very upset about the fact that I'm separated. I can't face up to it; I can't even talk about it. I'd rather pretend it never happened; I don't feel that there's a place in society for a woman who's so inhibited and separated too. Sometimes I don't know whether to say I'm married or separated. It's all so distressing that I can't even think about ever living with anyone again.

Dr Detinis: Why not?

Patient: I feel completely selfish, I can never give in over anything. Also because things aren't going at all well for me at the moment. I've stopped believing in anyone, in men, that is.

Dr Detinis: Why?

Patient: Well, I've always felt a bit like that about men, but getting separated made it worse. I had idealised marriage so much; mine lasted three and a half years and it was awful.

Dr Detinis: Why was it awful?

Patient: We just had totally different attitudes, though I didn't realise that at first. Neither of us could accept how the other one thought or behaved. We both tried as hard as we could to humiliate each other. And that actually seemed to make it harder to preserve what little self-esteem I have.

Dr Detinis: So would you say that you've always had a fixed concept of men, which on the one hand makes it difficult for you to have relationships, and on the other has an adverse effect on your self-esteem?

Patient: Yes, for instance, I think that men are always sexist, and women are always forced into certain roles. If a woman is very talented and intelligent then people say she's like a man; but if instead she stays at home and does the housework and looks after the children then she's a second-class citizen. And it's impossible to strike a balance between the two positions ('Envy'(39/II)). That's how I feel, at any rate. I've never been able to find a middle way. I've gone to both extremes; first I was a housewife who stayed at home, and then suddenly I rebelled against this and wanted to do other things; I couldn't combine the two. I found it quite impossible; before I knew where I was I had changed roles completely.

I realised that men are much better off, because society values men above women, and that's something I find hard to accept. For instance, I don't think men are sincere. When I meet men who seem nice, I partly want to get to know them better, but as soon as they find out what I'm like, it's all over. They think I'm impossible. I don't think a man could ever understand me because men are totally different to women. However hard I try to explain, they still judge me. I feel very inferior and I can't stand it.

Dr Detinis: What else can you tell us about your character?

Patient: I think that there are two sides, two faces, to me. On the one hand I'm very submissive, and on the other I'm completely the opposite. I'm extremely aggressive and difficult to handle. I always think I'm right and the other person is wrong; I always try to get my own way. At first I'm submissive, and then I show myself in my true colours, or else I start on an aggressive footing, as though I were expecting an attack. If the other person doesn't try to get at me then I calm down, but if he does I blow my top and the other side of me stays hidden. If they treat me like a normal person then that doesn't happen, but they hardly ever seem to. If they don't just judge me by my face or the mood I'm in, then I do behave normally, but I'm always ready to attack.

Nothing can stop me when I lose my temper, I couldn't care less if I hurt anyone or get hurt myself. Afterwards of course I feel very guilty and have to apologise to the other person or accept their apologies too, but if they throw them back in my face, if they don't understand, then that's it! I just don't want to know! I might go on thinking about them but I wouldn't have anything to do with them.

Dr Detinis: And how do you feel about them then?

Patient: I get upset and angry about the lack of understanding, and I also feel annoyed with myself because I couldn't keep control. I think perhaps I didn't explain everything properly, or I just got fed up with them ... I invariably feel as though I was the one who was mis-understood, but on the other hand I also think it was me who ruined everything. I seem to ruin every relationship and friendship I have.

I can't express my feelings either. For instance, when I'm depressed I feel irritable, but people don't notice that I'm depressed unless I'm in a very bad way, otherwise I'm almost always quiet and reserved. I haven't always been like that, I used to be quite communicative, but I've just become more and more reserved. Sometimes I feel as though I'll stay like that for ever. I find it so difficult to talk – to people of my own age, that is. I can talk to elderly people and children, though.

Dr Detinis: How do you get on with elderly people and children?

Patient: I show myself as I am. I can talk and sing, express myself as I am. When I'm with children I like to sing them songs, tell them stories, dance and skip about ... but I can't do that with anyone of my own age. With elderly people too I can talk about anything and feel comfortable and everything comes easily.

Dr Detinis: You said something about your emotions and about the way in which you relate to other people. Are you a loving person – what sort of things affect you or move you?

Patient: Children do. I love children, because I think they're the ones that need to be loved the most. I feel very sorry for children who don't get enough love and affection. You have to be prepared to spend a lot of time with them, you have to try to understand them and bring them up as best you can. That's when my best side comes out.

Another thing I like is travelling; there's a place called Jujuy, it moves me just to talk or hear about it. I love that place, I feel I've got roots there. I can identify with it because it's so far from civilisation. I like the fact that it's peaceful and very colourful; it's sad too, but I feel at home there. I like the people in Jujuy because they're gentle and natural and also because they don't talk much. I haven't ever lived there, but I've often stayed there for up to a month at a time.

I love that place. I love it when the people there are kind to me, though I could never tell them directly. Sometimes I think I should – I don't mean actually thank them, but just let them know how much I appreciate them. But I never do, I'm incapable of expressing anything like that, because I feel that if I did, the value of what I was giving would be lost. It's impossible to say what you feel, that's what I think at any rate.

Dr Detinis: A while ago you said 'I always think I'm right'. If the person with whom you're talking contradicts you, how do you feel?
Patient: It depends on how they say it. If they come right out with it and don't beat about the bush . . .

Dr Detinis: I mean an argument about anything; for example, if you think this ashtray is grey and they say it's black.
Patient: It depends – if I find the person interesting I'll forgive them, if not, then I'll argue with them.

Dr Detinis: What else can you say about your personality?
Patient: I'm very changeable. I swing from one mood to another very easily. I'm always like that. One moment I feel good in one place and the next I don't. Or I might be glad that I've got something and then suddenly I feel it's too much. ('Mood, changeable, variable, etc. (68/I)).

Dr Detinis: You said you're doing teacher training at the moment, and also working. What sort of work do you do?
Patient: I look after a 9-month-old baby.

Dr Detinis: Do you live alone?
Patient: No, with a family.

Dr Detinis: Do you have a family yourself?
Patient: Yes, but not here. I was born in Tandil.

Dr Detinis: And who lives there?
Patient: My mother and my brothers and sisters, everyone.

Dr Detinis: And your father?
Patient: He's dead. He died seven years ago.

Dr Detinis: What did he die of?
Patient: Cancer.

Dr Detinis: How many brothers and sisters have you got?
Patient: Three.

Dr Detinis: Older or younger?
Patient: I'm the youngest.

Dr Detinis: Why did you come to Buenos Aires?
Patient: Because of work. I used to work at the tourist resort in Tandil, and one day the lady I'm with now asked me if I wanted to come and look after her baby. We spent three weeks at the tourist resort in Cordoba and then came here.

Dr Detinis: When did you get married?
Patient: In 1979.

Dr Detinis: Was there any reason why you didn't have children?
Patient: I didn't want to get involved in something as complicated as that. On the one hand I did want to because I love children, but on the other I didn't because I knew it would have been awful for them to grow up with parents who were always at loggerheads. I didn't want them to suffer.

Dr Detinis: Was the marriage an unhappy one all the time?
Patient: Yes, right from the beginning. It was OK – but not good – for a month, not more than that. Then I started to get terrible nervous attacks and bouts of depression. I was on medication for about a year and a half.

Dr Detinis: What did you do, how did you react, when you felt depressed?
Patient: I used to cry a lot, alone of course, because I don't like people to see me crying. I always feel as though I'm being scrutinised.

Dr Detinis: How did it feel if someone came and offered you some sympathy or some advice when you were depressed . . . ?
Patient: There was an older lady whom I knew, she came almost every afternoon to see how I was . . . She was the only one. It did me good. I was living alone in Berazategui and she was on her own too, and she almost always came to keep me company.

Dr Detinis: What can you tell us about your childhood, about how you got on with your family, what you liked to do, what your hobbies were, what you do now, and what your plans for the future are.
Patient: I loved both my parents very much, but that was when I was very young. Most of all I liked animals, I still do in fact. I only ever played with them. We lived in the countryside, and I used to run off into the fields to play with the animals. And when I was older . . . I was happiest up to the age of five. I found it terribly hard to have to start going to school and meet other children. The school was near where I

lived and I used to run back home, I didn't realise that I had to stay there. That's when I started to have trouble getting on with boys. I've almost always been the same, anxious on the inside and aggressive on the outside. I used to fight with all the boys . . . I used to compete with them. I don't think I had any hobbies, but I was always fond of music. I think I would have liked to dance, and to draw too.

Dr Detinis: Why did you say 'would have liked to'?

Patient: Because I never did; I dance in my own way, and always on my own because it's something very private. I feel good when I'm dancing because I can express everything ('Dancing' (17/I)).

Dr Detinis: Are you a tidy person?

Patient: Yes, very, but there's a drawer that I like to put my hand into and mess things up.

Dr Detinis: And in the rest of the house?

Patient: I like to feel that I can put my hands on anything when I need it. I'm pretty obsessive about cleanliness; but I feel that to keep a house clean and tidy is to respect it properly ('Conscientious about trifles' (16/I)).

Dr Detinis: What are your periods like?

Patient: They come more or less every twenty-eight days and they last for four or five days.

Dr Detinis: How do you feel when you have them?

Patient: For the last year or so I've felt very depressed and irritable before they start, and I also get stomach cramps and nausea.

Dr Detinis: Which illnesses have you had?

Patient: The usual ones that children get – measles, mumps . . . When I was little I had a lot of problems with my ears, I got a perforated eardrum in my left ear when I was about a month old. I always had earache until I had an operation on my nose and throat when I was eleven. And then when I was older, perhaps eighteen, there was something wrong with my thyroid gland, the right lobe was inflamed or something like that. And about three years ago I had three cysts in the left ovary and two in the right. I haven't had any illnesses apart from that.

Dr Detinis: How does the weather affect you?

Patient: I don't like the weather here in Buenos Aires, it's so hot and humid. It wears me out and makes me feel nervous. I don't like humid or cloudy places.

Dr Detinis: What happens when it's cloudy?
Patient: I get depressed ('Cloudy weather agg.' (1348/II)).

Dr Detinis: Do you always feel depressed when it's cloudy?
Patient: Yes, except for when it rains; I love it when it rains hard.

Dr Detinis: Do you like the sun?
Patient: I love the sun.

Dr Detinis: Storms too?
Patient: Yes, they don't frighten me at all, I think they're really glorious – Nature in all her splendour. Most people are afraid of being struck by lightning, but I think it would be a very nice way to die. Much more natural than dying in your bed.

Dr Detinis: How do you feel when you're by the sea?
Patient: I get depressed by the sea, it's so boring just to sit there. There's the constant humidity too, and the salt water's bad for me.

Dr Detinis: What is your favourite food?
Patient: Pasta, roasts . . .

Dr Detinis: Do you like animal fat?
Patient: Only in small quantities.

Dr Detinis: Sweet things?
Patient: Jams and jellies; but not puddings made with milk.

Dr Detinis: Salt?
Patient: No, hardly any.

Dr Detinis: Spices?
Patient: If they're not too strong.

Dr Detinis: Bitter or sour things?
Patient: Bitter no, sour, yes. I like grapefruit, lemon tea and lemonade.

Dr Detinis: Milk?
Patient: Yes.

Dr Detinis: Eggs?
Patient: Yes.

Dr Detinis: Fish?
Patient: Fairly.

Dr Detinis: How hot do you like your food and drink?
Patient: I like my coffee and tea very hot; I might have an occasional soft drink in the summer, but I don't drink anything apart from that.

Dr Detinis: How do you take your tea in the summer?
Patient: Hot.

Dr Detinis: Have people remarked about it?
Patient: No, because I think it's normal.

Dr Detinis: What if it cools down a bit?
Patient: Then I wouldn't drink it, I don't like it tepid. If I had to I would, but I wouldn't enjoy it.

QUESTIONS FROM THE FLOOR

Question: You said that you don't drink much. Could you say why, please?
Patient: I don't drink much in winter, I don't like water or soft drinks . . . I drink lots of coffee and tea, but not water by itself. Sometimes in summer I have a soft drink.

Question: What would you like most to be?
Patient: Do you mean in an ideal or a real sense?

Question: What would you like to do?
Patient: I'd like to travel, make pottery and be able to dance well. I'd also like to be less shy.

Question: How did you get on with your mother and father?
Patient: As a child I got on well with my mother; I could talk to her until I was twelve or thirteen, but not after that. She was as aggressive as me. I always got on well with my father. He didn't show his affection openly, but there was a feeling of mutual understanding and respect. My mother couldn't understand me and she didn't give me the love I needed, like my father did.

Question: Why did you use the word 'respect'?
Patient: I don't think that my mother respected me as an individual; she was rather authoritarian in her relationship with me. My father was always aware of me, he didn't impose himself on me. He knew what I was capable of and didn't insist on my playing the role of dutiful daughter.

Question: What about your brothers and sisters?
Patient: I've got two sisters and a brother. I got on well with my brother. We used to fight a lot but we were both alike.

Question: How were you alike?
Patient: In our attitude and behaviour. I could relate to him when he felt upset. He was aggressive too but I knew he had problems and

didn't express them, except indirectly, by behaving badly or being surly. I realised that he was like me and I understood him. He's a lovely person – I think he has good feelings but he doesn't know how to deal with them.

Question: You said you take your drinks very hot. Are they literally boiling hot, or do you let them cool down a bit?
Patient: I let them cool down a bit.

Question: What does travel mean to you?
Patient: Going away, seeing new places. I like the idea of feeling that a place does and doesn't belong to me at one and the same time, if you see what I mean. I suppose I just feel really free, really at home in some places.

Question: Would you say that travelling is a way of filling a void in you?
Patient: Yes, you could put it that way.

Question: How do you sleep and what do you dream of?
Patient: I feel tense when I sleep because my arm and my shoulder-blade hurt, and I wake up feeling tired. In the last few months I've almost always dreamt that I was arguing with my family.

Dr Detinis: Have you had a recurring dream throughout your life?
Patient: Twice I dreamt that my cat in Tandil had been killed and I was terribly upset. (*Cries*)

COMMENTARY

I hope that everything the patient said has stayed in your minds, because this is a beautiful example of a remedy expressed in its essence. Let us examine all the aspects of the case, from childhood onwards, and see what symptoms emerge.

Here is a patient whose behaviour and expression mirror what she says she feels. She is depressed and apathetic, irritable and aggressive. She spoke from first to last in a dreary monotone, and her emotional state remained unchanged, except at the end. Her inexpressiveness is telling.

Since her childhood she has been able to form bonds only with animals; one may thus deduce that she has not managed to form relationships with other people. And that is the problem which she brings here: her difficulty in relating to other people. She cannot integrate herself and therefore cannot make friends or form a stable relationship. She said, 'I seem to ruin every relationship and friendship I have'. She cannot form bonds; that is her existential predicament. Since childhood she has lived in isolation, as she does now. 'I can identify with Jujuy because it's so far from civilisation . . . I like the people there because they don't talk much.'

She has the symptom 'Indifference, loved ones, to' (55/I), despite claiming to be a loving person. Reading between the lines, we can see that there are contradictions; at times we must deduce the symptoms rather than take them literally. The point to note about this apparent contradiction is that she cannot give. She said, 'I find it very hard to give because I feel as though nothing I can give is worth anything', and 'I feel very selfish, I can never give in over anything'. Earlier she had said, 'I find it hard to get on with people'.

Two fundamental aspects of the remedy are this emotional indifference and her inability to relate to her femininity. She said that she competed with the boys at school and for this reason could not integrate. Her marriage broke up after three and a half years: 'We had totally different attitudes' and 'We both tried as hard as we could to humiliate each other'. 'Men are always sexist . . . if a woman stays at home and looks after the children then she's a second-class citizen'. 'Society values men above women, and that's something I find hard to accept'. This is her conflict. 'First I was a housewife who stayed at home, and then suddenly I rebelled and wanted to do other things' . . . 'I feel very inferior to men and I can't stand it'.

At the beginning she said, 'I do what I think I ought to and not what I want to'. This symptom is 'Will, contradiction of' (95/I). A closely related symptom is 'Undertakes things opposed to his intention' (91/I), but in this case the more general rubric applies.

This woman is Sepia. Sepia is obsessed with cleaning and polishing, she is the star of all those advertisements for detergents and soap powders. If her husband or the children do not take their shoes off when they come in, they soon catch the sharp edge of her tongue. She is meticulous, demanding, a perfectionist. This symptom, which she expressed very clearly, is 'Conscientious about trifles' (16/I). Its emphasis varies from remedy to remedy. It has some of the elements of obsessional neurosis; for example, the presence of a locus of disorder within an otherwise pristine environment.

Strictly speaking, we are straying from the bounds of homoeopathy here, but this will help us to understand the symptom. The patient said, 'There's a drawer in which I keep everything jumbled up'. This drawer is the place in which, so to speak, she keeps disorder itself. In purely homoeopathic terms, it is her mania for cleanliness which is of value to us.

'Envy' (39/II), in this case of men, is a vital symptom. Many women are Sepia from birth, but one cannot identify the remedy until they begin to confront the feminine aspects of their character. They will often fall ill after having children, because they reject these qualities in their competition with men. Lycopodium women compete directly with men in everything, but principally intellectually, because culturally men are considered superior to women. Sepia, on the other hand, is competitive for much deeper reasons, and specifically with regard to her sex. She is in conflict with her femininity.

Sepia women are not usually sterile, at least no more so than any other remedy, and many of them have lots of children. They are, however, often emotionally cold and have a low libido.

Another symptom is 'Manipulative', which does not appear in the repertory. The patient said, 'I always try to get my own way'. Lycopodium is dictatorial, but Sepia is manipulative.

Other symptoms which the patient has are: 'Mood, changeable, variable, etc.' (68/I), 'Cloudy weather, agg.' (1348/II), and 'Company, aversion to' (12/I). No remedy shuns other people as much as Sepia does. Her isolation is pathetic, and she may go so far as to take to her bed and lie there in complete darkness so that no one should come in and disturb her solitude.

REPERTORISATION

'Indifference, loved ones, to' (55/I)
'Company, aversion to' (12/I)
'Envy' (39/II)
'Will, contradiction of' (95/I)
'Mood, changeable, variable, etc.' (68/I)
'Cloudy weather agg.' (1348/II)

Prescription: Sepia 10M.

Index of Remedies

Aconitum Napellus, 2, 26, 61, 75
Aesculus, 61
Agaricus, 9, 26, 95, 113
Agnus Castus, 61
Alcohol, 107, 109
Aloe, 82, 95
Alumina, 13, 47, 53, 116
Ammonium Carbonicum, 61, 104
Anacardium, 15, 31, 54, 89
Anantherum, 37, 87
Angustura, 31
Antimonium Crudum, 15, 107
Antimonium Tartaricum, 16
Apis Mellifica, 61
Argentum Nitricum, 25, 61
Arnica, 16, 31, 43, 53, 77, 98
Arsenicum Album, 23, 32, 61, 74, 81, 88, 96, 107
Asterias Rubens, 54
Aurum, 10, 13, 31, 36, 61, 62, 111

Baryta Carbonica, 95
Benzoicum Acidum, 45
Borax, 8, 9, 82
Bovista, 38, 77
Bromium, 82
Bryonia, 16, 32
Bufo, 17, 40, 82

Caladium, 18
Calcarea Acetica, 16, 53
Calcarea Carbonica, 16, 53, 55, 61, 62, 95, 98, 102, 167, 200, 202
Calcarea Fluorata, 85
Calcarea Phosphorica, 36, 81
Calcarea Sulphurica, 53
Camphora, 99, 101
Cannabis Indica, 95
Cannabis Sativa, 59, 77

Cantharis, 82, 84
Capsicum, 20, 77, 88, 99
Carbo Animalis, 60, 62, 68, 69, 99, 111
Carbo Vegetabilis, 60, 61, 77
Carboneum Sulphuratum, 25, 36
Carcinosin, 39, 102
Carlsbad, 23, 68, 109
Castoreum, 53
Causticum, 38, 53, 54, 61, 82, 99, 101, 109, 113, 114
Centaurea Tagana, 68
Chamomilla, 2, 20, 21, 77, 85, 96, 99, 104
Chelidonium, 13, 99
China, 44, 61, 75, 81, 82, 83, 96, 107, 110
Chininum Sulphuricum, 53
Chloralum, 25, 40, 88
Cicatrin, 188
Cicuta Virosa, 16, 71, 77, 94, 96, 104
Cina, 28, 53, 77, 82, 107
Clematis, 53, 55, 68
Cobaltum, 13
Coca, 40, 82, 85
Cocculus, 13, 18, 79, 82, 88
Coffea Cruda, 107, 110
Coffea Tosta, 9, 111
Colocynthis, 98
Comocladia, 92, 104
Copaiva, 94
Corallium Rubrum, 28
Crocus, 9, 26, 77, 88
Crotalus Cascavella, 26, 42
Crotalus Horridus, 77, 94
Cubeba, 8, 18, 60, 77, 85, 113, 118
Cuprum Metallicum, 38, 85
Curare, 47, 48, 60, 77, 94, 118
Cyclamen, 13, 16, 28, 55, 94, 108

Index of Rubrics

CLASSICAL HOMOEOPATHY
Dr Margery Blackie
Edited by Dr Charles Elliott and Dr Frank Johnson
360 pages, 216x138 mm, 1986, Repertory Edition 1990
ISBN 0906584140

This book sets before the reader the enthusiasm, learning and deep clinical understanding of one of the foremost homoeopaths of our time.

Classical Homoeopathy draws into one volume Dr Blackie's teaching over the whole span of her career. The first part describes the thinking behind homoeopathy and the principles on which the successful homoeopathic prescription is based, with its recognition of the sick person as a body, mind and spirit relationship, bound inseparably as one. The major constitutional remedies are then studied in detail, either individually or differentiated within groups of related remedies. This is followed by the symptomatic treatment of illness or disability, analysing each of the remedies that may be of value, and distinguishing the particular circumstances in which one remedy is likely to be indicated in preference to another. Next there is a compact materia medica, summarising the essential characteristics of one hundred and eleven major remedies. The final part comprises a clinical repertory, relating symptoms to remedies already discussed in the book, and an index of remedies.

'It is an essential book for all those with a genuine interest and belief in homoeopathy, for it reveals so clearly Dr Blackie's incomparable style of practice and knowledge of materia medica. However, the complete beginner will be swamped with so much fact, and would be wise to delay purchase for a short time until they have gained a working knowledge of homoeopathy. Thereafter, the book will be invaluable.' *Homoeopathy*

EVERYDAY HOMOEOPATHY
Dr David Gemmell
184 pages, 216x138 mm, 1987. ISBN 0906584183

This book shows you how to use homoeopathic medicine in the everyday context of your own personal and family health care. It covers the problems that the lay person is quite likely to have to cope with, either as first aid or else in a wide variety of complaints and disorders that may not be urgent but where relief and cure are sought.

The author starts by describing the thinking behind homoeopathy, its stress on the need to assess the patient in his or her entirety as an individual, and its freedom from toxic side-effects. There is the necessary basic information on how to observe symptoms and select a remedy, as well as on potency and dosage.

The main part of the book is presented in four sections – accidents and first aid, the problems of women, children's problems and general problems. The author explains the nature of each problem and suggests common-sense measures to be taken whatever else is done. He then discusses the various personal circumstances and particular symptoms that may be present, using these to point to the appropriate homoeopathic self-treatment.

He highlights the cases where self-help is out of place and medical advice must be sought without delay. He also highlights the cases where homoeopathy can provide a more complete and effective cure, but where self-help is equally inappropriate and a professional homoeopathic evaluation must be obtained.

'For years now my patients have been asking me what the best book is to help them understand how they can use homoeopathy for their family. I have always been uneasy about the books I've had to recommend because they always seem to fall short of the ideal. . . . At last someone has written this book, and it comes across as the work of a thorough, caring, down-to-earth physician who knows just what he is talking about.' *Holistic Health*

HOMOEOPATHIC PRESCRIBING
Dr Noel Pratt
87 pages, 216x120 mm, revised edition 1985. ISBN 0906584035

This book is written for all who use homoeopathic remedies. Clear indications are given wherever it is important that the lay person should also obtain medical advice.

One hundred and fifty-six common complaints and disorders are covered in the book, arranged alphabetically. A selection of appropriate remedies is then listed, together with details of the particular symptoms and signs that enable the prescriber to differentiate between each of them. There is an appendix on the constitutional types. The book is printed with interleaved blank pages, to enable the reader to amplify the text on the basis of personal experience.

'Dr Pratt has written a very useful vademecum for those with a good working knowledge of homoeopathy. The way the book is set out makes for clarity and ease of access to the appropriate information.' *Homoeopathy Today* (UK)

HOMOEOPATHY AS ART AND SCIENCE
Dr Elizabeth Wright Hubbard
Edited by Dr Maesimund B. Panos and Della DesRosiers
344 pages, 216x138 mm, 1990. ISBN 0906584264

Dr Elizabeth Wright Hubbard was one of the most brilliant homoeopaths of the twentieth century. This book represents a large part of her teaching and writing, setting before the reader her great gift of being able to describe homoeopathy in a way that imprinted itself in the minds of all who studied with her.

She begins by examining the nature and philosophy of homoeopathy and its relationship with conventional medicine. This is followed by a discussion on the use of the repertory and then by a major section on remedies, in which she displays her wide-ranging and often intuitive mastery of the materia medica. There is a further major section on cases, demonstrating the skill with which she was able to match the symptom picture of the patient to the proved indications of the relevant remedy. The final section of the book comprises the famous 'Brief Study Course in Homoeopathy'. Here she explains in expanded detail how the homoeopath proceeds in the evaluation and management of the individual case.

'What a treasure trove this book is, a posthumous collection of essays from one of the most brilliant homeopaths of the twentieth century. . . . They are perhaps the most pleasurable way for someone schooled in allopathic thinking to grasp the essence of the homeopathic mind. They illustrate the idea of the simillimum, the minimum dose, and the single remedy in a way which mentioning these principles here does nothing to convey. . . . They are essentially anecdotal evidence and they are essential reading. When the inadmissible evidence has been disclosed we have learned the truth.'   *Homeopathy Today* (USA)

HOMOEOPATHY IN PRACTICE
Dr Douglas Borland
Edited by Dr Kathleen Priestman
208 pages, 216x138 mm, 1982, Symptom Index Edition 1988
ISBN 090658406X

Dr Borland presented this material as a course during the 1930s at the London Homoeopathic Hospital. His homoeopathic insight remains as fresh and as valuable today as it ever was.

The book is divided into two sections. The first, entitled 'Homoeopathy in Clinical Conditions' deals in turn with injuries and emergencies (including acute pain), headaches, sore throats, respiratory and heart conditions, obstetrics and gynaecological conditions, sleeplessness, and pre- and post-operative conditions. The second section, 'Studies and Comparisons of Remedies', shows to what extent Dr Borland excelled in the way he led from one remedy to another, often linking them by their differences or similarities. He first looks at six Kali salts, and then at five Natrum salts, all well known to the homoeopathic prescriber. 'Seventeen Important Remedies' are then discussed, and a comparison made between three more – Lilium Tig., Natrum Mur. and Sepia. The final chapter deals with the use of four nosodes – Psorinum, Tuberculinum Bovinum, Medorrhinum and Syphilinum. A remedy index and a symptom index complete the work.

> 'The book comprises some fourteen chapters, nine devoted to a study of various clinical conditions, and five to studies and comparisons of remedies. Even when the conditions are common and we all have to deal with them daily, the treatment is fresh and there are unusual angles on well known remedies and interesting comparisons on smaller remedies.'
> *The Homoeopath*

INSIGHTS INTO HOMOEOPATHY
Dr Frank Bodman
Edited by Dr Anita Davies and Dr Robin Pinsent
119 pages, 216x138 mm, 1990. ISBN 0906584280

The purpose of this book is to show that it is possible to subject homoeopathy to the same standards of intellectual scrutiny that apply to any other branch of medicine.

The author begins by explaining this specialty as it first confronts the conventionally-trained mind, and follows with an analysis of the extraordinary contribution made by its founder, Dr Samuel Hahnemann, to modern medicine. There are several chapters on the use of homoeopathy in psychiatry, in which Dr Bodman had much experience. He then discusses the homoeopathic management of a wide variety of clinical conditions, including allergy – the area where research during the 1980s has demonstrated the effectiveness of the microdose. He concludes with a discussion of the reasoning that lies behind research into homoeopathy.

> 'The possibility of achieving a lasting cure is squarely counterpoised to the palliative aim of much orthodox drugging. . . . It is clear that the author has not just read, but studied and considered carefully the meaning of Hahnemann's writings.'
> *The Homoeopath*

INTRODUCTION TO HOMOEOPATHIC MEDICINE
Second Edition
Dr Hamish Boyd FRCP
285 pages, 216x138 mm, 1989. ISBN 0906584213

This book provides a systematic introduction to the principles of homoeopathic medicine. It shows how the homoeopath's selection of a remedy is based on a process that goes beyond the diagnosis of a particular condition to a perception of the patient as a whole and individual person.

The homoeopathic materia medica is discussed in relation to the systems of the body and the patient's presenting complaints, in a framework that will be familiar to any doctor. The author uses this framework to describe the subsequent management of the patient in homoeopathic terms. He describes the clinical conditions in which homoeopathy is particularly useful, and those where conventional treatment is likely to be necessary, as well as the circumstances where orthodox medicine and homoeopathic medicine can fruitfully be used in conjunction with one another.

The symptom pictures of fifty-five of the most important remedies are then described in detail, offering the reader a sufficient basis on which to introduce them into his or her own practice. Dr Margaret Tyler's valuable 'Study of Kent's *Repertory*' is given as an Appendix.

> 'The book is clearly laid out and well presented. The material is divided into clearly defined chapters which make it easy to dip into. I felt it succeeds well as an introduction to homoeopathic medicine, presenting the material simply. but at the same time leaving nothing out. I liked particularly the way in which Dr Boyd expressed the importance of utilising the best of homoeopathic medicine and the best of orthodox medicine. He got the balance just right.'
>
> *The Homoeopath*

MATERIA MEDICA OF NEW HOMOEOPATHIC REMEDIES
Dr O. A. Julian
637 pages, 216x138mm, 1979. ISBN 0906584116

This book offers a rich collection of over a hundred new homoeopathic remedies. It adds to existing knowledge, supplementing the classic materia medicas. Some of the remedies are completely new. Others are familiar substances used homoeopathically for the first time. Most of them have been the subject of a Hahnemannian proving, while the remainder have undergone a clinical symptomatological study and their value has been confirmed in therapeutic use.

A detailed clinical repertory is provided at the end of the book, together with an index of clinical keynotes. Principal symptoms are italicised throughout the text. There is a bibliography for each remedy, as well as chemical information of pharmaceutical relevance.

'Dr Julian must be complimented on beginning the reappraisal of the existing materia medica for the late twentieth century, and for introducing in critical fashion so many new remedies.'

Homoeopathy

STUDIES OF HOMOEOPATHIC REMEDIES
Dr Douglas Gibson FRCS
Edited by Dr Marianne Harling and Dr Brian Kaplan
538 pages, 216x138 mm, 1987. ISBN 0906584175

Homoeopathic remedies come from every part of the world and from all the kingdoms of nature – mineral, vegetable, animal and microbe. They include strong poisons such as arsenic, the venom of deadly snakes and the products of disease, as well as harmless substances like sand and charcoal, and herbs whose healing properties have been handed down through generations and are celebrated in history and legend.

Dr Douglas Gibson was a distinguished homoeopath who recognised the importance of knowing the materia medica in depth. These studies of remedies, first published in the British Homoeopathic Journal over the period 1963–1977, combine the panorama of each remedy with a faithful description of the mental and physical symptoms it elicits from a sensitive prover. The whole remedy is indeed used to treat the whole patient.

His studies are edited here for publication in book form. They differ from any previously published materia medica in the uniquely wide range of insights that are brought to bear on each remedy. They will be of great practical value, and a source of pleasure and stimulation, to the homoeopathic clinician.

'This is a classic text in which author, editors and publishers have proved equally worthy of each other. It will assist the neophyte and established homoeopath equally in becoming more competent and reliable prescribers.'   *British Homoeopathic Journal*

TUTORIALS ON HOMOEOPATHY
Dr Donald Foubister
200 pages, 216x138 mm, 1989. ISBN 0906584256

This book offers the reader an insight into Dr Foubister's clinical experience, gained over a long career in homoeopathic practice. His writings are remarkable for the extent of his knowledge and his close attention to detail.

The contents reflect many of his particular strengths. The first section studies the factors that underlie the homoeopath's evaluation of the individual patient. This is followed by a section of several chapters on paediatrics, in which he excelled. There is then a comprehensive section on Carcinosin – his development of the Carcinosin remedy picture was his major contribution to homoeopathy and it gained him worldwide acclaim. He then discusses a number of other remedies in detail, with a final section on specific conditions. The book ends with an Appendix of therapeutic hints that had served him well.

'Dr Foubister has managed in masterly fashion to compress his immense knowledge of virtually the whole field of this fascinating discipline, encompassing his life experience in clinical research with special reference to his own particular expertise in paediatrics.'   *Homoeopathy Today (UK)*

TYPOLOGY IN HOMOEOPATHY
Dr Leon Vannier
Translated by Dr Marianne Harling
176pp, 246x189mm, 1992. ISBN 0906584302

Typology, the classification of human beings according to their physical and psychological characteristics, is as old as medicine itself. It is particularly relevant to those forms of therapy which take account of the whole person. Dr Vannier attached great importance to the subject, believing that it could help the homoeopath to know the patient better, and the patient to perceive more clearly the full extent of his or her own potential.

He takes as his models the gods of Antiquity – Mars, Saturn, Apollo, Venus, Jupiter, Mercury, Luna and Terra – studying their mythological attributes as prototypes of the mental and physical characteristics of human beings. Each of these principal types is described at length under the following headings: physical make-up, morphology, intellect, character, the conditions and problems to which they are prone, and the changes that are likely to occur with age and circumstance. He then studies in detail the homoeopathic remedies to which the individual types respond best – usually a group of six to eight related remedies dominated by a major polychrest.

Dr Vannier makes it clear that no human being is a pure prototype, exhibiting one set of characteristics alone, and that in his view two, three or even four types will be found in one person, either together in varying degree, or else in succession. He describes briefly a number of 'metatypes' – combinations of prototypes – which he names after gods not included in the original eight.

The text is illustrated throughout with line drawings and photographs, showing how artists and sculptors from classical times until the present century have depicted the different types and their many variations.

'This work is the mature achievement of one of the acknowledged masters of French homoeopathy. . . . I feel that it can be of real help to any homoeopath seeking to get beyond the over-simplistic idea of treating the individual. Between our unique individuality and our common humanity are all the complex groups to which we belong: sex, age, race, nation, class, temperament, psychological type and so on. Our troubles arise from the conflicts and misunderstandings between these, not from our humanity or our uniqueness. So it is opportune that this excellent, readable translation of Vannier's classic should appear in English. May it stimulate thought and observation rather than slavish satisfaction that the system is a complete one.'

British Homoeopathic Journal

'*Typology in Homoeopathy* is a unique, information-packed book which is off the beaten path of our collection of materia medica texts. It is a reference book which is easy to enjoy and yet, if studied in detail, can broaden our knowledge of the human condition.'

Resonance (USA)

HERBAL MEDICINE
Dr R. F. Weiss
Translated by A. R. Meuss
362 pages, 246x189 mm, 1988. ISBN 0906584191

Herbal Medicine is the English translation of the current Sixth Edition of *Lehrbuch der Phytotherapie*, a book which has established itself as an indispensable modern text in the field of medical herbalism. This latest edition takes full account of present-day research findings, from which Dr Weiss has added many further suggestions for prescriptions, as well as indications for new areas of application.

The introductory chapters examine the nature of the subject and provide the necessary guidelines for prescribing. The main part of the book then studies the large and impressive body of plant drugs, arranged on a basis of clinical diagnoses relating to particular systems – digestive, cardiovascular, respiratory, urinary, nervous, female reproductive, the skin and the eyes. There are separate chapters on influenza and colds, rheumatic conditions, some metabolic and endocrinal disorders, the use of herbal medicine in cancer, the treatment of wounds and other injuries, and the therapeutic use of herbal baths.

In every case the relevant plants are discussed, with information on their occurrence and botanical features, differentiation from related species, constituents and medicinal actions. Many of them are illustrated by line diagrams. The treatment sections offer a wealth of suggested prescriptions, with details of dosage, application and precautions. Where appropriate, proprietary formulations are also included. Full references are given throughout. There is a comprehensive subject index of almost two thousand entries.

'It is refreshing to have in English an established practical work from the hands of a senior medical practitioner who has used herbal remedies for over six decades. . . . The strength of this book is in its appearing like a written account of an apprenticeship with a master craftsman: that alone will make it compulsory reading for anyone interested in using herbal remedies well.'

Complementary Medical Research